THE FROM SCRATCH RHYTHM WORKBOOK

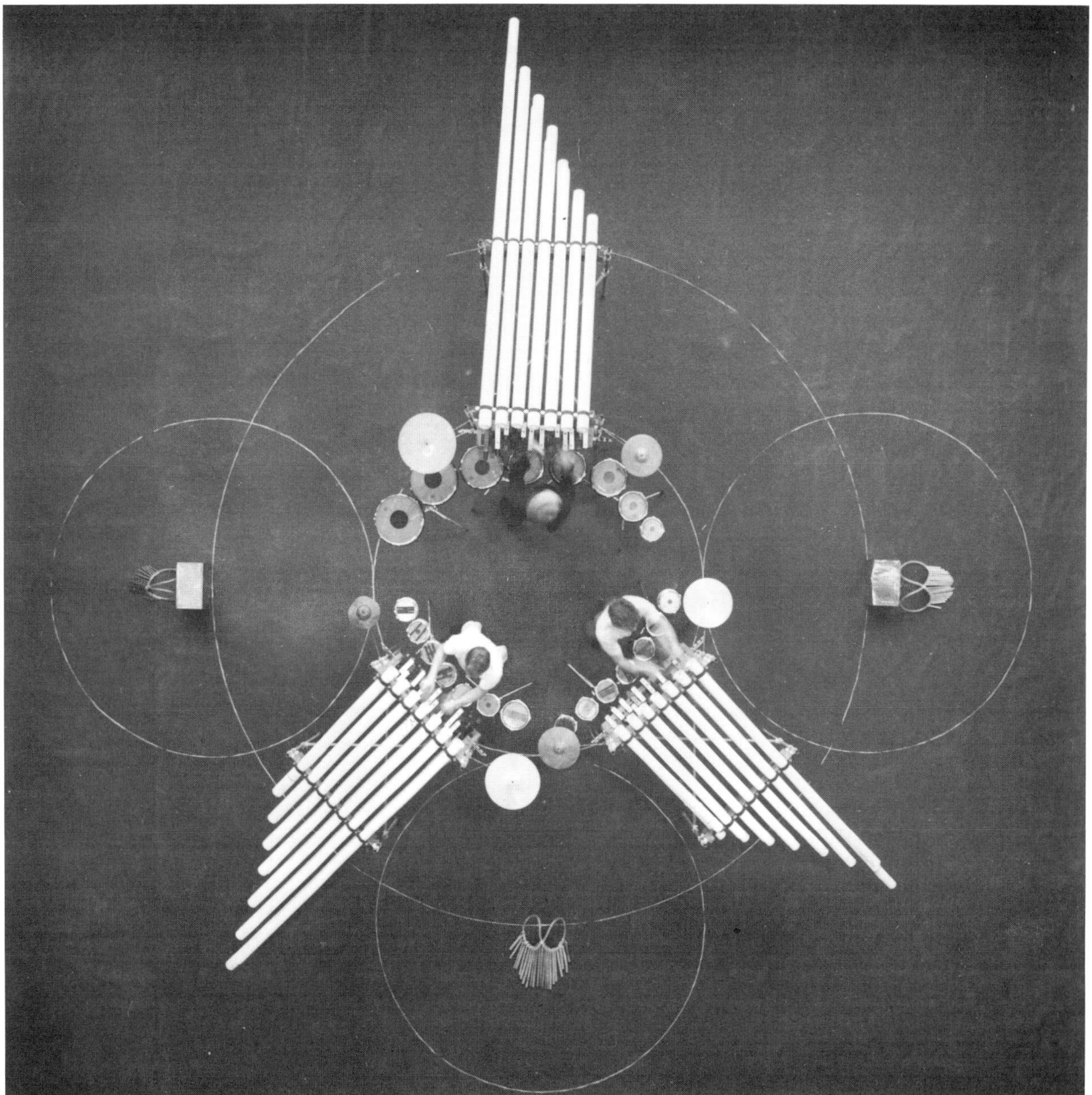

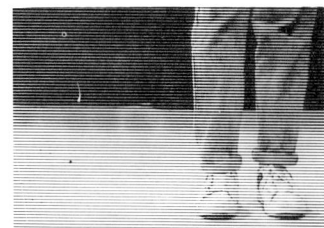

WALLY FLOYD

THE FROM SCRATCH RHYTHM WORKBOOK

by
Philip Dadson
Don McGlashan

Heinemann
Portsmouth, NH

123171

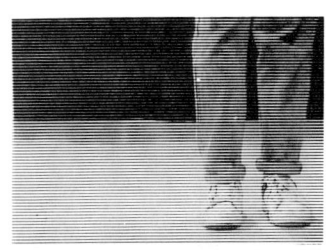

Heinemann
A Division of Reed Elsevier Inc.
361 Hanover Street
Portsmouth, NH 03801-3912

Office and agents throughout the world

Copyright © 1990 by Philip Dadson and Don McGlashan
Copyright © 1995 by Philip Dadson and Don McGlashan

All rights reserved. No part of this book may be reproduced in any form or by any electronic or mechanical means, including information storage and retrieval systems, without permission in writing from the publisher, except by a reviewer, who may quote brief passages in a review.

We would like to thank those who have given their permission to include material in this book. Every effort has been made to contact the copyright holders for permission to reprint borrowed material where necessary. We regret any oversights that may have occurred and would be happy to rectify them in future printings of this work.

Editor: Lisa Barnett
Cover Design: Julie Hahn

Library of CongressCataloging-in-Publication Data

Dadson, Philip.
   The From Scratch rhythm workbook / Philip Dadson and Don McGlashan.
     p.   cm.
   Discography: p.
   Includes bibliographical references
   ISBN 0-435-08670-7
   1. Musical meter and rhythms—Studies and exercises. 2. Musico-callisthenics. I. McGlashan, Don. II. From Scratch (Musical group)
MT32.D33F7 1995
781.2'2—dc20   95-10195
                                                                            CIP
                                                                             MN

Printed in the United States of America on acid-free paper
98 97 96 95   VG   1 2 3 4 5 6

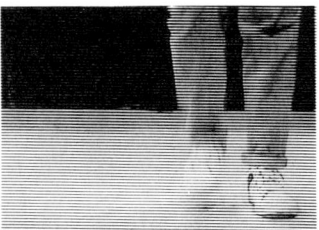

CONTENTS

Introduction v
    Notes for Classroom Teachers ix

1. Call and Response 1
2. Walking in a Circle 5
3. Hocket Game 8
4. Birthday Piece 1 11
5. Birthday Piece 2 14
6. Random Pulse 1 and 2 16
7. Odds and Evens 18
8. Stamping 1 22
9. Stamping 2 24
10. Ostinatos and Solos 26
11. Pulse and Improvisation 1 29
12. Ons and Offs 1 32
13. Ons and Offs 2 37
14. Ons and Offs 3 39
15. Pulse and Improvisation 2 41
16. Action Loop Games 43
17. Combination 1 46
18. Combination 2 50

Appendixes
1. A Glossary of Common Rhythm and Musical Terms 57
1A. A Guide to Understanding the Musical Notation in This Book 58
2. Vocal Warm-ups 62
3. Developing On/Off Singing 66
4. Composing Rhythms: A Few Ideas 69
5. VOM (Variable Occasion Music) 1972 71
6. Some Instrument Ideas 87

From Scratch *Recordings* 102

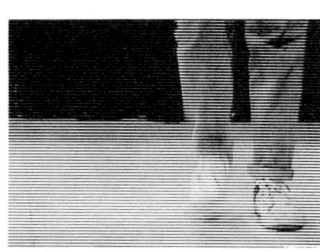

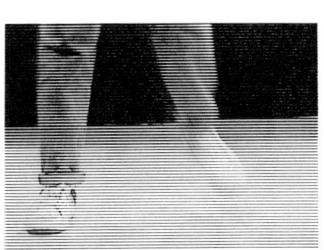

INTRODUCTION

Exploring rhythm and sound and searching for new tones with found or homemade instruments is enjoyed the world over. There is an old Sanskrit saying, "Rhythm is the father of life and tone the mother." When they join they make music and the whole world dances.

This book aims to expand knowledge and enjoyment of rhythm and sound. It is designed equally for individuals who want to develop their own musical skills and for any group of trained and untrained musicians and performers, actors, dancers, students—in short, anyone who will benefit from a body-based approach to rhythm.

From Scratch is a New Zealand group formed in 1974. Returning to basics, the group began by experimenting with sound and form in musical and visual ways, using homemade instruments and simple repetitive rhythms. Over time, *From Scratch* music has increased in complexity. Its densely textured rhythms form the core of lengthy works that are part music, part theatre, part ritual, and part sculpture, and although the music has evolved, it remains based on the same rhythmic language with which the group began.

During this time many simple exercises have evolved. These are used regularly in rhythm workshops and in warm-ups for live performances, and have gradually gelled into the "game" forms you will find in this book. The exercises and games are graded, beginning with the simplest and leading to the more difficult. Instructions are set out in easy-to-follow stages so that a teacher or workshop leader can easily absorb the concepts for practical use—or in the case of a music or performing group, so that members can readily "apply and try" in the course of a rehearsal or warm-up. (Where two games using similar concepts are listed, the second is usually more demanding, but also more interesting.)

Using these exercises regularly (as we do within *From Scratch* and in rhythm workshops), we find that everyone is soon achieving at a similar rate.

We have emphasized a body-based approach to rhythm—clapping, stamping, simple vocals, etc.—but all the exercises and games can also be adapted to work with musical instruments.

We hope that you will feel free to use this material as a basic resource, adapting and extending exercises to fit your specific needs. Also, by using the exercises in this book as ingredients to be mixed together and developed creatively (as in *Combinations 1 and 2*), you can devise new group rhythm works that are both challenging to perform and effective for an audience. We hope you are led to some new and exciting results.

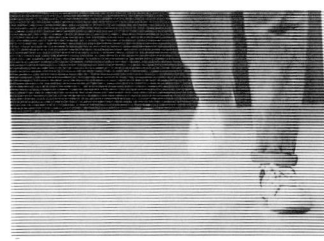

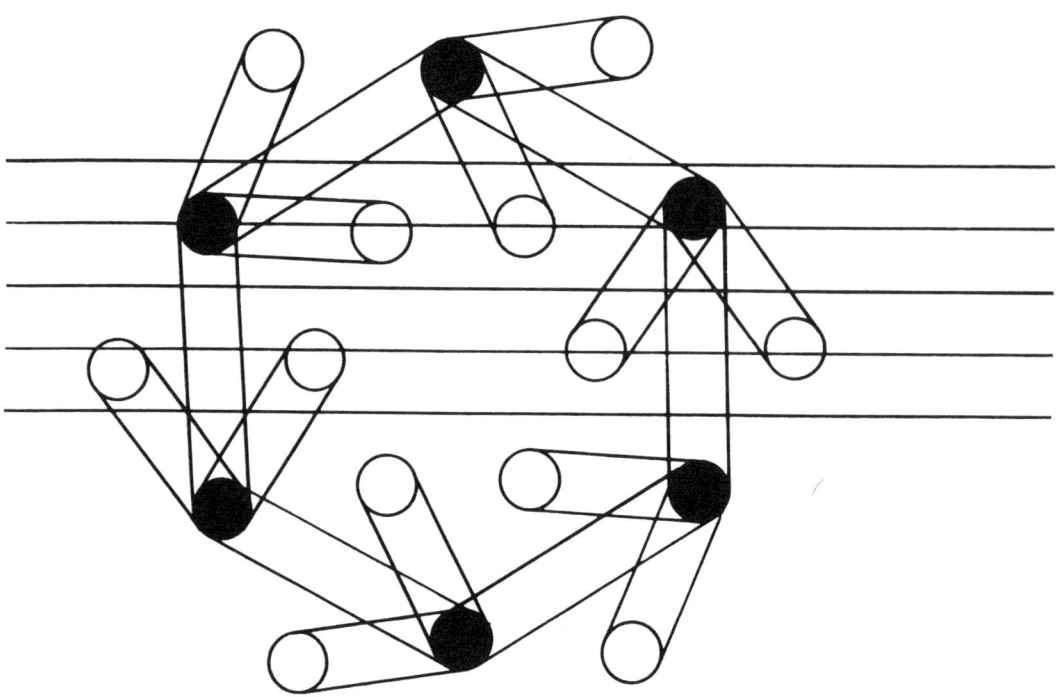

Notes for Classroom Teachers

If working with rhythm is new territory for you, have no fear. Any new language takes a little time to figure out and part of our aim is to familiarize you with this language via the games and exercises in this book.

We suggest you spend some time with the first game, titled *Call and Response*. The instructions are detailed and will help you come to grips with our description style and with the simple musical notation that we use occasionally to illustrate rhythmic ideas.

Our approach to rhythm, as described earlier, is body-based, with foot stepping, hand-clapping, and simple vocals. When movement is described, try it out. It's usually easier than you may imagine.

The footstepping patterns are universals. They (or variations of them) are used in folk traditions all around the world. Derived from walking and natural work rhythms, they help to get the pulse firmly grounded in the body, as well as being a simple and effective device for keeping time.

Sometimes, presenting a movement to a class for the first time can have its difficulties, but there are ways around this. Find out in advance what kinds of street and dance music rhythms your students enjoy and/or what simple footstepping patterns they may use in their own cultural traditions and go through some of these with the group, explaining their function in terms of time

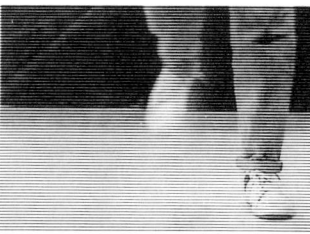

keeping. Some of their movements may well form the basis for adaptations to the exercises we suggest. In essence, be flexible and open to improvisation.

The musical notation we use is basic. Think of it as a kind of shorthand that has been developed over the centuries to streamline the playing and writing of music. It saves a lot of complicated written instructions. If notation is a first time experience for you, Appendix 1A explains it all.

The space in which you perform these games and exercises is important. The floor area should ideally be large and clear—the floor surface wooden, linoleum, cork, or similarly tiled. Concrete tires the limbs and carpet tends to absorb any feet sounds. Classrooms are multipurpose and can usually be arranged to accommodate mild physical activity, but if yours can't, try booking the gymnasium or any similar open space you can find. Entrance halls and courtyards are often ideal and underutilized.

Clothing and footwear are also worth a mention. Loose-fitting clothes and light shoes or sportshoes are best. The exercises in this book range from mildly physical to vigorous, and while they primarily aim to be a fun method of learning, they also keep you fit.

Teachers, once they are familiar with the various games and exercises in this book, should feel free to experiment with the order of the exercises in ways that best suit the requirements of their groups. It is also worth mentioning that while short, intensive workshops can cover a lot of ground, the best results with this material are achieved from 30- to 60-minute sessions on a regular basis.

If you have any queries, comments, or suggestions concerning this book, don't hesitate to contact us. And if as a result of exploring these ideas you devise a new rhythm game or exercise, please let us know. We'd like to hear from you. Send details to, *From Scratch*, P.O. Box 66060, Beachhaven, Auckland 1310, New Zealand.

Good luck!

Phil Dadson/Don McGlashan
for *From Scratch*

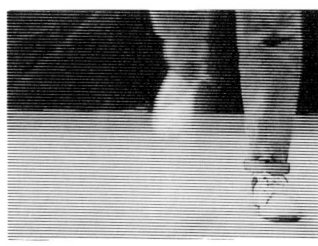

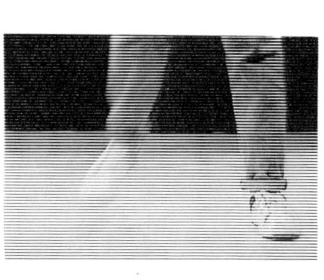

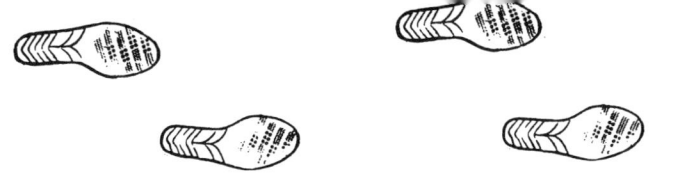

1 CALL AND RESPONSE

Background

Rhythm, while it is part of the language of music, is also a language of its own, and there is no better way to learn it at the outset than by imitation. This game follows a "call and echo" format to get everyone clapping and later vocalizing often intricate rhythms "by ear."

The first foot-stepping pattern introduced here is basic to many games and exercises that follow. Its function (like a simple dance pattern or marching) is to set up a reliable body pulse that keeps the group together but leaves everyone's hands and minds free for other things like clapping and vocals. Once everyone relaxes into it, the foot pattern plays the same role of group timekeeper as a drummer in a rock band or a conductor in an orchestra. This idea is common in music and dance traditions all around the world.

All of the following games and exercises need to be "counted in," and it's useful to have a consistent method that everyone can use for getting things started. The count-in must be in the same speed relationship as the game you are about to perform. The basic beat should be established first with a finger click or handclap, and then the game is counted in as follows.

```
         ♩    ♩    ♩    ♩  | ♩    ♩    ♩    ♩   START
COUNT    1,        2,       | 1,   2,   3,   4
```

Activity Sequence

1. Get the group in a large circle facing inward. Demonstrate the basic side-to-side foot stamp. Count steadily and slowly:

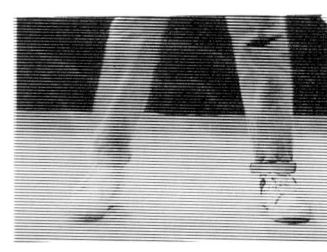

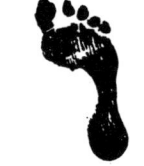
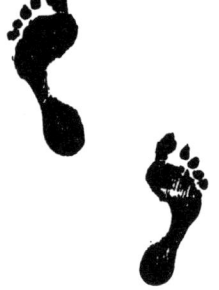
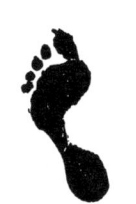
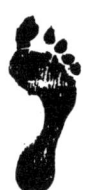

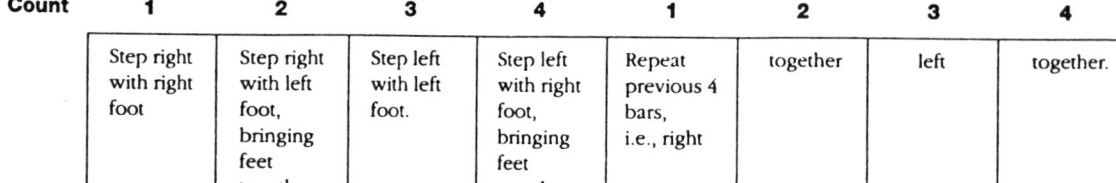

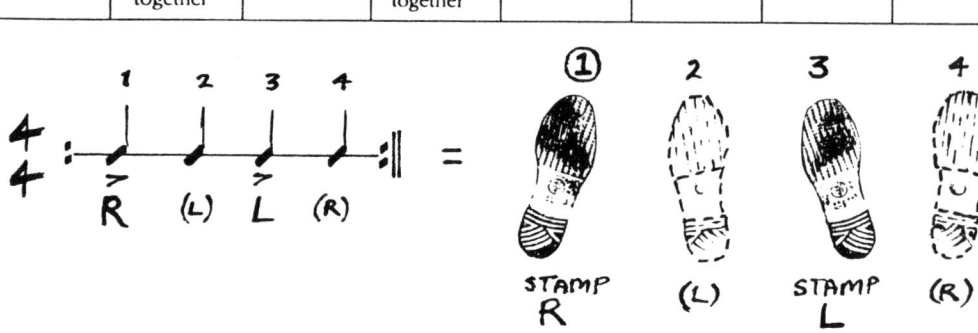

Legs should be slightly bent, the upper body straight but relaxed and arms free to swing naturally. Try and make it as natural as walking. A pulse about ♩ = 120 works well to start with. Let everyone get comfortable with it before proceeding onto 2. (If you are in any doubt about this, flick the pics in the bottom corners of the pages.)

2. The basic clapping game is based around a cycle of four beats that are synchronized with the side-to-side foot stamp. The sequence in four stages is passed from one player to the next and goes like this:

Call A	Starting on the right foot, the leader claps four regular beats in unison with the foot pulse pattern.
Response	The rest of the group imitates.
Call B	The leader improvises a rhythm based on the four beats.
Response	The rest of the group imitates the rhythm.
Call C	The leader improvises another rhythm different to the first.
Response	The rest imitates.
Call D	The leader improvises a third and last rhythm different to those previous.
Response	The rest imitates, and then the role of leader passes to the next on the right who repeats the sequence from A to D.

Explain and run through this a few times until it's clear. The notated example illustrates *one possible* sequence. (If musical notation is new to you, see Appendix 1A for a simple guide to understanding notation basics).

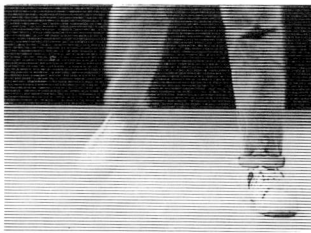

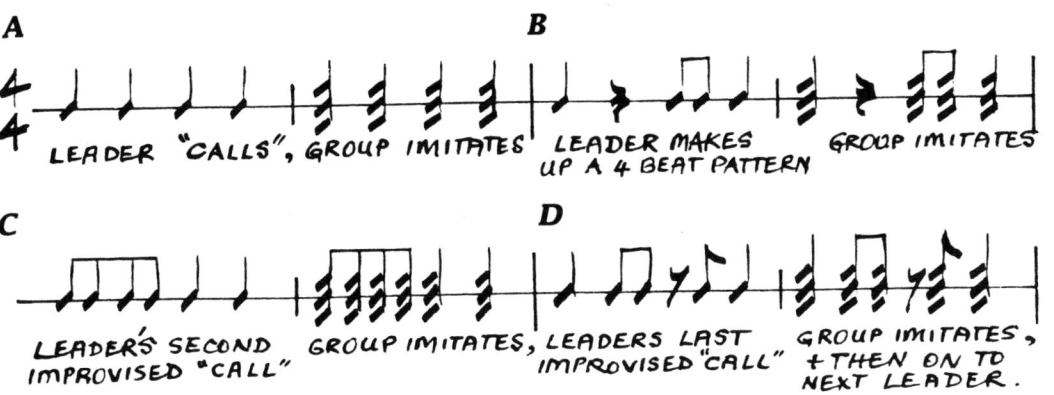

Points to note

- The first "call" for each new leader should be:

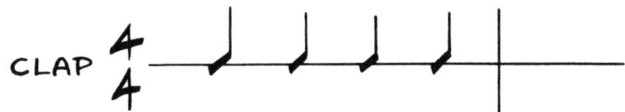

    (This gives everyone a chance to get their bearings.) The remaining three calls are up to them.

- Calls should not take longer than 1 bar of 4/4, nor start before the downbeat.

- Don't make your improvisation so clever that you lose your foot pattern.

- Rests are effective but everyone has to count them accurately.

    Now start the game off going continuously around the circle with the role of leader always passing to the right. When everyone has been leader, start a new game as follows (and it's good to keep the foot pattern going while you explain things).

3. In this version, each leader has only 3 calls to make, and all 3 can be improvised—or the first call can still be as in (A). To make things more interesting, try introducing some body percussion and vocals—sung sounds, shouts, words, etc.—as well as clapping.

    After the leader has made the third call, she has to point to someone in the group who becomes the next leader. If she forgets to point, or is too late, the flow is interrupted and she has to solo again. This helps build group cohesion—you have to watch the person who's soloing, because you may be next! (Be prepared to prompt the pointing a bit until the idea is established).

    When this is going well, start allowing the foot pattern to speed up. See how fast the group can get before the piece disintegrates.

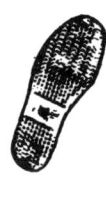
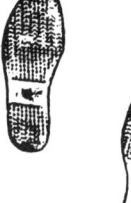
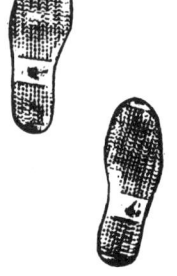

Developments

4. Get the group jogging in a circle and do the same two call/response games (2 and 3), but this time use only voice sounds instead of clapping. It doesn't have to be melodic. Whoops, whistles, and yells are fine as well. People tend to be less inhibited by now because they know the structure of the game and they're doing something physical at the same time. The pointing game can get pretty fast and furious here, and it's very good for group connection, rhythmic, and listening skills, as well as being a great warm-up and a lot of fun.

5. Once the group has the foot-stepping pattern running on auto, try version 1 again, but this time fitting two claps to each foot pulse. The four basic beats of the clapping cycle now match two beats of the foot pulse cycle. The foot pulse is in half notes and the clapping is in quarter notes.

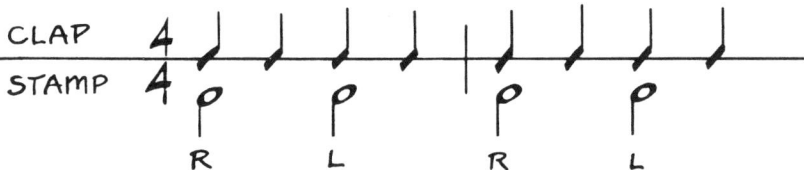

This gets easier with practice and will eventually make the performance of the games and exercises more relaxed physically. You can now do the foot stepping at *half* the previous speed. (Try *Birthday Piece 1* to get this well established.)

Points to note and/or discuss

1. If the group is large, follow 2 steps: (1) divide up into two circles and run the two simultaneously, making sure the foot-stepping of both groups is in unison first. This sounds good as well as focuses the concentration within each group. (2) Shorten the number of cycle repeats in stage 1 to three, and in stage 2 to two, so that things move along a little faster.

Advanced exercises

1. Try all of the preceding exercises using basic units of 3/4, 5/4, and 6/4. (The foot step should not change, just the accents.) This is difficult, so be patient.

2. Try exercise 2 and/or 3 using gestures instead of sounds, or a combination of claps, voice, and gesture. Keep movements and gestures to the upper part of the body only, so the foot pulse is not interrupted. Tricky patterns with the feet invite chaos.

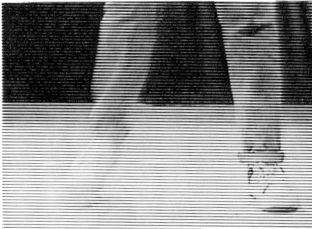

2 WALKING IN A CIRCLE

Background

Many of the exercises in this book are linked to some kind of whole-body movement in an attempt to introduce the idea that our bodies are, in fact, organized rhythmic systems containing many different cycles (pulse, breathing, eating, sleeping, etc.). The way we use our bodies in everyday life is rhythmic, too. When we walk, run, swim, work, etc., our bodies are executing steady, reliable, and very musical rhythms, whether or not we are aware of them!

These walking exercises help to illustrate this point. They are also useful in introducing the idea of different-length cycles.

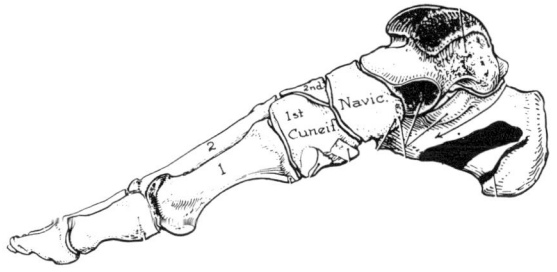

Activity Sequence

1. Get the group walking at their own natural speed in any direction around the space. Take this time to explain that walking is a cycle, and that each person's walking speed is unique to them. It has to do with the length of their legs, how much coffee they may drink, and many other factors.

    To make everybody aware of the complex set of body movements involved in an action as simple as walking, try slowing everyone's walk down to slow motion, and then back up to normal speed.

2. Get the group to gradually find a common direction (walking in a circle anti-clockwise around the room) and a common pulse (which will be the average of everyone's walking speed). Allow time for the group to adjust so that everyone is in step. The movement should be relaxed, i.e., not marching or stamping.

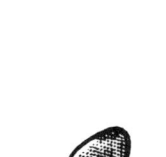

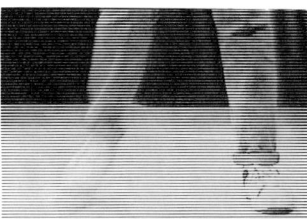

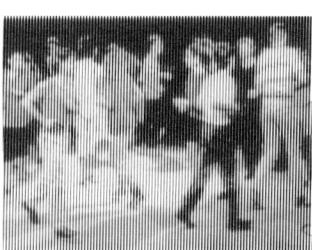

3. Continue walking in step, in a circle, and get the group to stamp with their right foot on the 1 of an 8-step cycle:

$$\frac{8}{4} \; \underset{\underset{1\ \ 2\ \ 3\ \ 4\ \ 5\ \ 6\ \ 7\ \ 8}{\overset{>}{R}\ \ L\ \ R\ \ L\ \ R\ \ L\ \ R\ \ L}}{\Big\| \; \downarrow\ \downarrow\ \downarrow\ \downarrow\ \downarrow\ \downarrow\ \downarrow\ \downarrow \; :\Big\|}$$

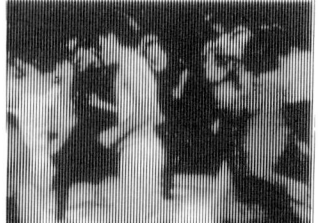

4. Then on the 1 of a 4-step cycle:

$$\frac{4}{4} \; \underset{\underset{1\ \ 2\ \ 3\ \ 4}{\overset{>}{R}\ \ L\ \ R\ \ L}}{\Big\| \; \downarrow\ \downarrow\ \downarrow\ \downarrow \; :\Big\|}$$

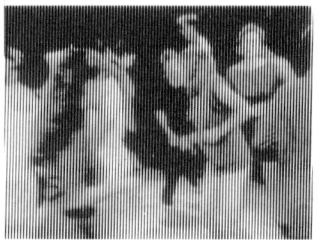

5. Then on the 1 of a 5-step cycle, noticing how the accents alternate between right and left:

$$\frac{5}{4} \; \underset{\underset{1\ 2\ 3\ 4\ 5}{\overset{>}{R}\ L\ R\ L\ R}}{\Big\| \downarrow\ \downarrow\ \downarrow\ \downarrow\ \downarrow :\Big\|} \underset{\underset{1\ 2\ 3\ 4\ 5}{\overset{>}{R}\ L\ R\ L\ R}}{\Big\| \downarrow\ \downarrow\ \downarrow\ \downarrow\ \downarrow :\Big\|}$$

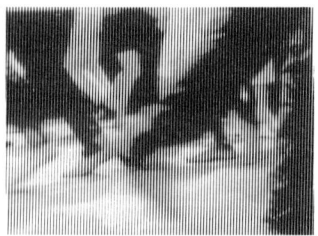

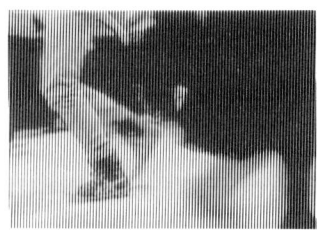

6. Make this left-right alternation stronger by getting the group to angle the right stamp *out* of the circle and the left stamp *in*.

7. Now make a longer piece out of different-length cycles. Repeat the 4-step cycle four times, then without stopping, change to the 5-step cycle, also repeated four times. Continue in this way through a 6-step cycle, a 7-step cycle, and finally an 8-step.

$\frac{4}{4}$	R L R L	R L R L	R L R L	R L R L	$\frac{5}{4}$
	$\overset{>}{1}$ 2 3 4	② 2 3 4	③ 2 3 4	④ 2 3 4	

$\frac{5}{4}$	R L R L R	L R L R L	R L R L R	L R L R L	$\frac{6}{4}$
	$\overset{>}{1}$ 2 3 4 5	② 2 3 4 5	③ 2 3 4 5	④ 2 3 4 5	

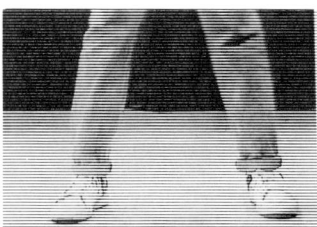

Practice this with the group until the ideas are firmly established. Start the process by counting out loud as follows:

One two three four, *two* two three four, *three* two three four, *four* two three four, *one* two three four five, *two* two three four five, *three* two three four five, *four* two three four five, etc.

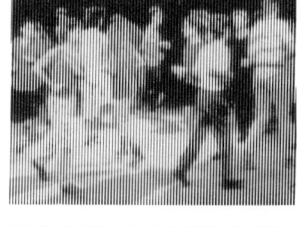

Add a shout on each stamp (initially the spoken "count" will do, but aim to get everyone *feeling* the cycle lengths rather than counting out loud).
   Try using a high vocal sound for a right stamp, and a low one for a left stamp. (Make sure that the pulse doesn't speed up. Encourage everyone to relax and feel the way in which their own body weight is carried along by the group pulse.)

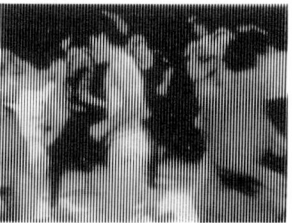

8. Try the same exercise, this time going all the way from four 1s to four 8s.

9. Now try *reversing* the exercise, starting with 8s (again repeated four times), working backward through 7s, 6s, etc., all the way down to 1s.

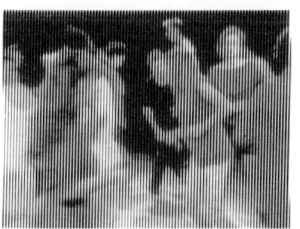

Developments

1. Now divide the group in two. Make two circles, one inside the other, going in opposite directions. The outside group starts with four 1s, then four 2s, and so on, finishing at the end of the fourth 8.
   The inside group does the opposite, starting with four 8s and finishing with four 1s. If you start everyone together, and you all keep to the pulse, you should end up with a piece that is interesting both to listen to and to look at. (And with luck, everyone should finish together!)

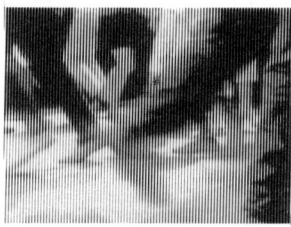

2. Try a seamless run in both directions: with the outside group going from 8s down to 1s, then 1s back up to 8s—and the inside group going from 1s up to 8s, then 8s back down to 1s. For added excitement, try including a rapid change of direction at the center point.

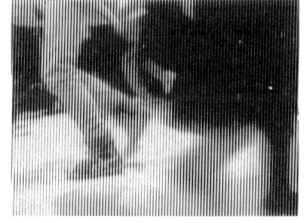

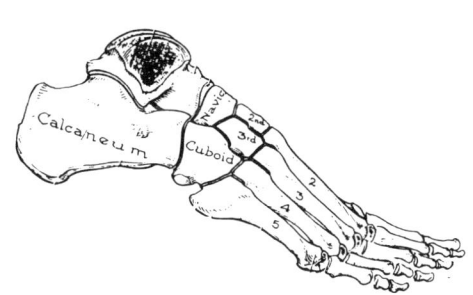

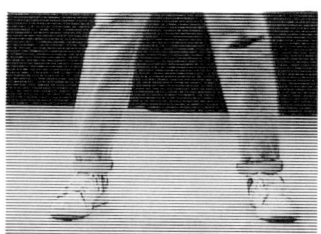

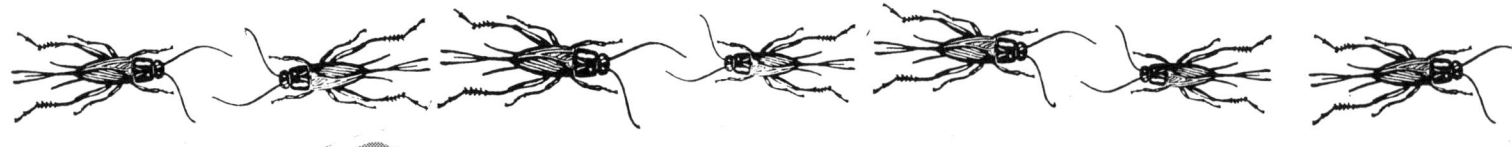

HOCKET GAME

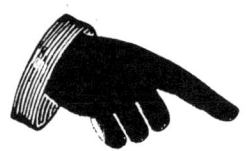

Background

"Hocketing" is the sharing of a rhythmic and/or melodic line between two or more players, one part having a rest when the other has notes. While the name "hocket" comes from medieval music, the style is still found all over the world wherever there is rhythmic group music-making.

This game involves a rotating conductor's role and gets everyone fitting individual bits into a larger and regularly changing rhythmic texture. The general aim is to make interesting and flowing hocket rhythms, i.e., repeating (and layered) rhythms composed of sequences of individual and often quirky sounds.

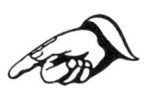 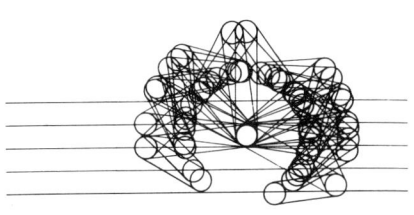

Activity Sequence

1. Form a large circle. Get everyone doing the side-to-side foot stamp at a nice easy pace, around ♩ = 76, and explain the following:

    - Everyone gets a short vocal or body percussion sound ready. It can be anything at all, a word, a grunt, a squeak, or whistle, or something musical. The "sound" should be short in duration and easily repeatable.

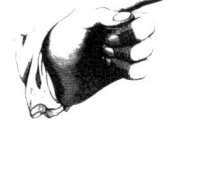

2. A "conductor" volunteers to stand in the center of the circle (still doing the foot stamp with the rest of the group). His first task should be to "sample" all the various sounds on offer, by pointing to everyone in turn (on the beat).

3. This done, the conductor's role is to point accurately on the beat (and off the beat once the procedure is well underway) to individual soundmakers—one after the other—so that a short repeating "rhythm" is established (3–5 sounds are a good start for a rhythm length).

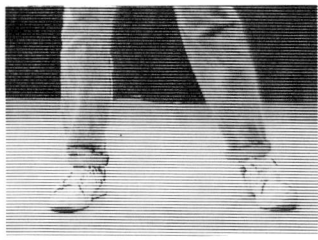 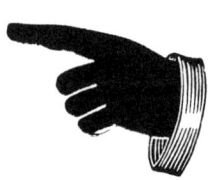

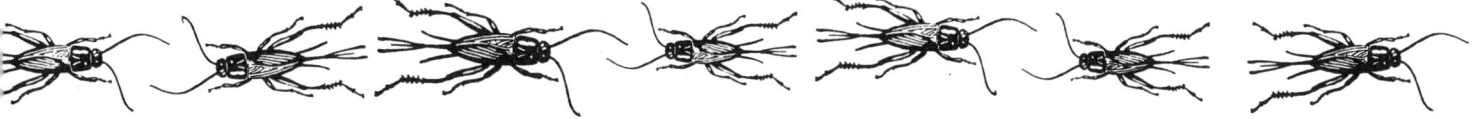

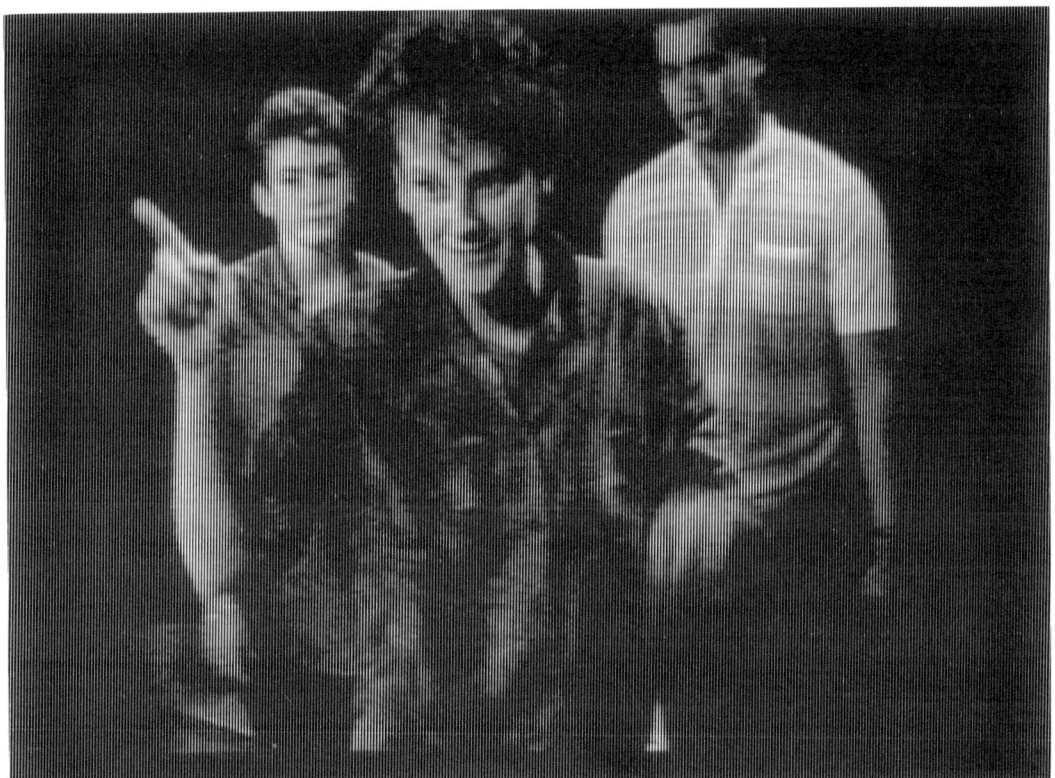

- For smooth running, a few hand signals are required for the conductor:
  a clear "point" for the benefit of the soundmakers
  a clear stop sign
  a "repeat till stopped" signal, a rotary movement of both hands
  a "volume control" signal, by raising or lowering both hands

- The soundmaker's task is to respond as quickly as possible to the cue from the conductor, and this can get pretty streamlined if the conductor is pointing accurately and the soundmakers are responding instantly.

- A sound should remain the same for as long as it is part of an active rhythm. Sounds can and should be changed between rhythms.

- The conductor can move from one rhythm to another without stopping, or layer rhythms on top of each other, or a combination of the two.

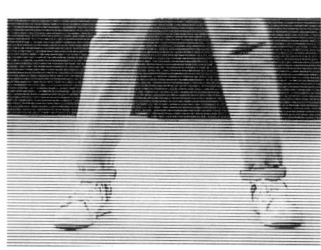

- To layer rhythm on rhythm, use the repeat till stopped signal to continue one rhythm while another or others are developed. The stop and volume signals may also be useful here.

- Change conductors after three or four successful rhythms have been completed.

Developments

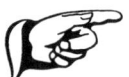

- If your group number is more than 10 to 15, establish two or more circles of around 8 to 10 per circle. This gives everyone a better chance to be conductor and makes the conducting role generally easier. Any one of each group can start out as conductor in the middle.

- Establish a common speed for the foot pulse to keep everyone in time. When there are two or more groups, this is important, and everyone will need reminding to keep an ear on the pulse.

- You might like to try this game using everyone's first name, with everyone saying their name or an abbreviation of it any way they like. Besides being word-based, it's also a good way of getting a group that is together for the first time on first-name terms.

Points to note and/or discuss

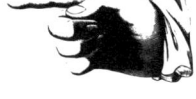

- What hocketing is, and how the role of the conductor can be minimized once a rhythmic pattern is established.

- How sounds can be generated to complement one another. Contrast in the sounds make for interesting rhythms and textures.

- A changeover of conductor usually occurs after a sequence of successful rhythms, but may also be prompted if a conductor defaults or stays in too long.

- When there are two or more groups, encourage everyone to be aware of the overall rhythm texture as well as being focused on their individual task.

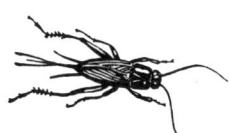
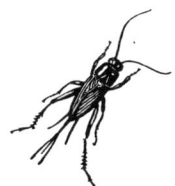
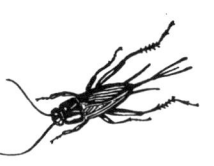
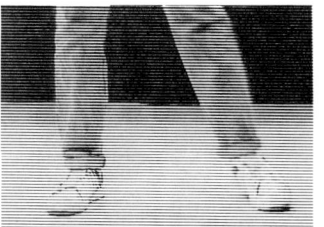

4 BIRTHDAY PIECE 1

Background

Every human being is an individualized world with complex internal rhythms and drives, but as social beings we also fit into groups as part of the larger world. In these games, ideas of the "collective" and the "individual" are combined and developed within the framework of one long cycle based on the highest even-numbered birthdate in the group.

These games are also very useful for introducing the skill of clapping and counting two beats to every foot pulse, i.e., thinking in terms of the foot pulse representing half-notes, and the clapping and counting, quarter-notes.

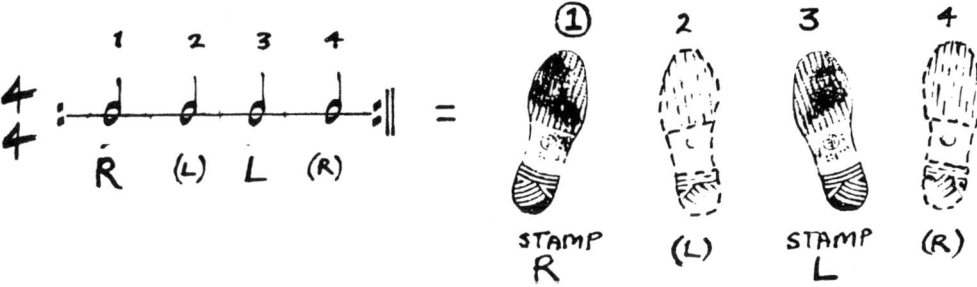

Activity Sequence

1. Get the group to form a large circle with everyone making the unison side-to-side foot stamp at a slow pace (about ♩ = 80).

2. While the group is getting comfortable with this "half-speed" stamping pulse, find out whose birthday falls latest in the month. When you've ascertained who's got the highest number, round it off (if necessary) to the nearest even number. This now becomes the whole group's cycle length.

   For example, if the highest-numbered birthday in the group is on the 29th, round it off to 30, and get the group to clap and count a 30-beat cycle (two counts to every foot stamp), with a big shout on the number 30 each time it comes around.

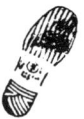
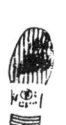

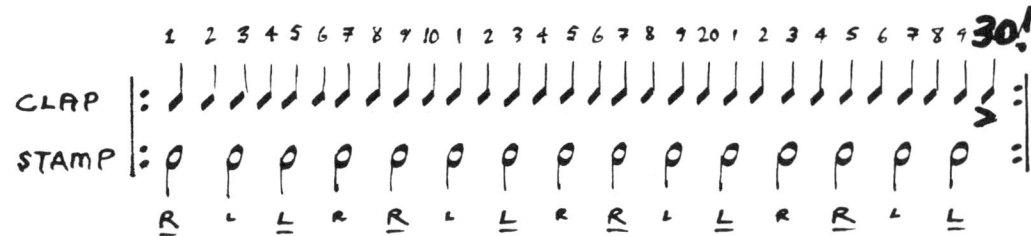

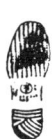

3. With everyone quietly continuing the foot-stamp pattern, you can explain the next stage. This involves everyone making a big sound every time their *own* birthday number comes around in the larger cycle.

They can begin by just shouting their own number; then, after a few cycles, using any loud yelp, whistle, or noise they want to make. If they can, they should accompany their sound with a big physical movement (but not with the feet, as it's important not to lose track of the foot stamp and the count of the larger cycle).

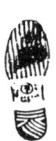

One or two people (probably the workshop leader and whoever's birthday number is highest) should be responsible for maintaining the long cycle into which everyone fits their exclamation.

Get everyone softly clapping the quarter-note beats over the half-note foot stamp. Once the long cycle is established and everyone is also accenting their own number within the cycle, give a signal to the group to stop the clapping so that the sound and gesture exclamations can pop in and out clearly.

Developments

4. After a series of the preceding cycles, get everyone, in their own time, to begin an independent cycle of counts based on their own birthday number. (That is, straight after an exclamation, each person begins counting again from 1 instead of carrying on to 30 or whatever.)

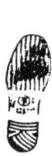

From this point on, their own birthday number becomes their new cycle length. Out of one large cycle many sub-cycles then evolve, still held together by the common foot stamp. As individuals move into their personal birthdate cycles, they are also now free to move anywhere inside or outside the circle, establishing their own "world" in relation to one another.

- Once again, the long cycle, with its accent on the last count, should be maintained throughout this stage by one or two people.

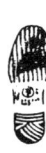

- Holding onto an odd-numbered cycle length over a slower pulse takes extra concentration, as accents will shift between the right and left feet, and will also regularly fall inbetween downbeats.

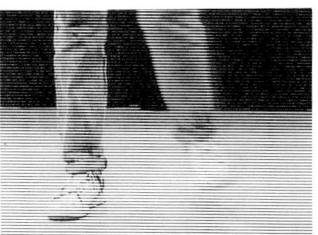

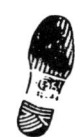

5. This final stage involves everyone's returning to the circle and the larger cycle in their own time, once again fitting their birthday number into the larger cycle with an exclamation as in stage 3. When all are back in, those counting the large cycle shout "last time" and everyone ends together on the end of the cycle.

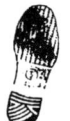

6. Try doing stages 3 through 5 in a continuous progression, making clear that the long cycle should remain consistent throughout, and should act as the anchor from which everyone should take their cue. (If the progression from one large cycle to sub-cycles and back again is difficult, try *Birthday Piece 2* and come back to this later.)

Things to note and discuss

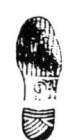

- How, in nature, rhythmic texture is the combined result of many different-lengthed cycles of sound. (Refer to the notes to *Random Pulse 1 and 2*.)

- How it's important to be able to make your exclamations without losing your focus in the larger cycle.

- How odd-numbered cycle accents shift between the left and right feet and inbetween downbeats. Being prepared for this will help.

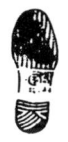

- Closing your eyes in stage 4 may help with focus. Some numbers, particularly the odd cycles, may need it.

- The lower numbers, 1 through 8, need good clear sounds, and 1, of course, becomes a quarter-note pulse reference.

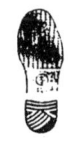

- In stage 5, if there's any difficulty returning to the larger cycle, stop, return to the circle, and resume as you pick up the count.

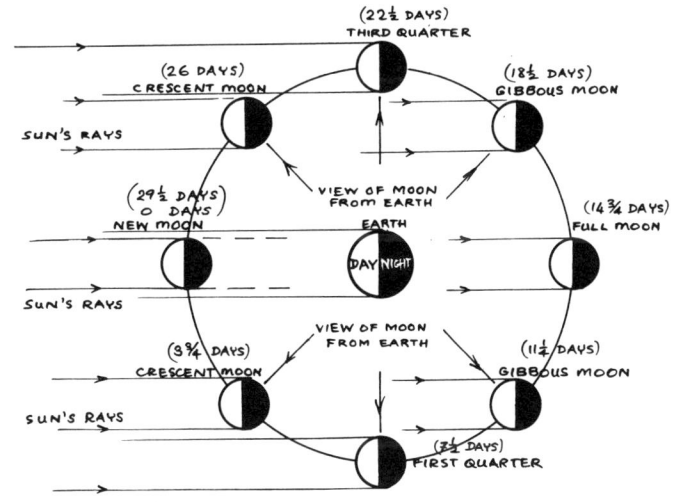

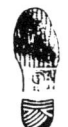

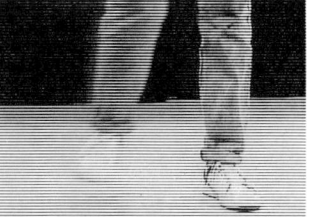

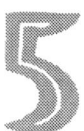 BIRTHDAY PIECE 2

Background

This exercise is another way into the ideas of *Birthday Piece 1*. As with many other exercises in the book, this can have the potential of developing into a small performable piece.

Activity Sequence

1. Get the group standing in a circle, facing in to the center and doing the side-to-side foot stamp (one beat per foot pulse, as in *Call and Response*).

2. Find out the day of the month on which each person was born (as in the previous exercise). Starting with the smallest birthday numbers, give each person one of the notes of a pentatonic scale to sing on the downbeat of their cycle. Use "ah" or a similar syllable.

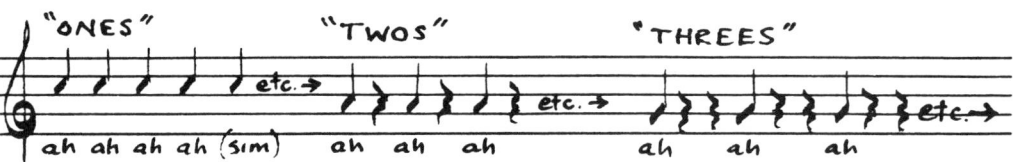

The smallest four or five numbers therefore become an "ostinato" on which to build the rest of the texture.

3. Now get those with larger numbers to invent their own notes or vocal sounds. These can get longer and more weird as the numbers get higher!

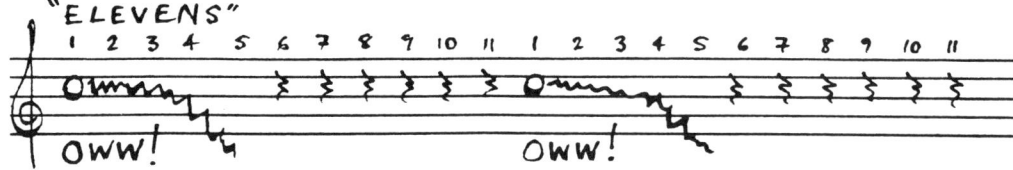

4. When everyone has learned their part, choose a conductor (as in the *Hocket Game*) who stands in the middle of the circle and brings parts in and out

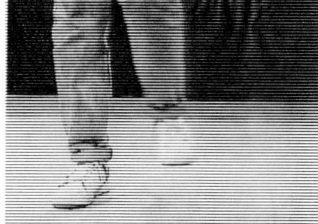

by using hand signals. It works well initially to start the piece off beginning with the smaller numbers and working up to the larger. Make sure the conductor allows each new part several repetitions to establish itself before the next part is brought in. (See "Points to Note and Discuss.")

Once all parts are sounding, have the conductor experiment with cutting out parts one by one, but in a different order from the build-up, until all parts are silent.

5. Get different members of the group to conduct/compose pieces out of this material, bringing parts in and out (one at a time or together) and indicating volume (both of individual parts and of the whole group).

Advanced exercises

As with all of these exercises, it's important that the whole group stays locked into the common foot-stamp pulse. Once the pieces are going well, however, it can be interesting, as a variation, to work without the foot stamp. This means that the interlocking ostinato parts become the timekeeper.

Points to note and discuss

In this exercise, and many of the others in this book, the individual "cells" or "cycles" are fixed, but the number of repetitions before the next entry is up to either the players or the conductor.

Music that contains repeating patterns that gradually evolve out of one another (sometimes called "process" music) often uses this method. The element of improvisation is not in the actual notes played, but in the decision of when to change to the next pattern. This is also a feature of much African and Polynesian drum music.

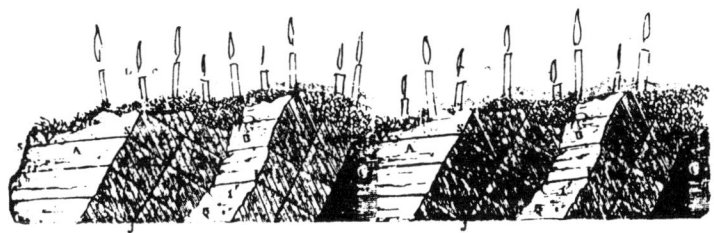

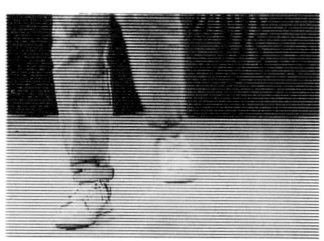

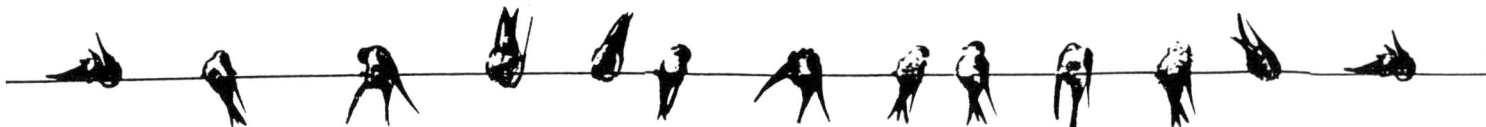

6. RANDOM PULSE 1 AND 2

Background

In our experience of nature there appear to be two main sorts of rhythm—the seemingly organized and the seemingly random. In the seemingly random the main effect is one of rhythmic texture, as in the collective sounds of insects and animals—a chorus of frogs, cicadas or crickets, a tree full of starlings, a zoo full of animals, a room full of people, and so on.

If, however, you isolate any one individual insect, bird, or animal and listen to it, you will hear a seemingly organized rhythmic pattern, often in relation to a pulse.

If you listen to any pair of singing insects, birds, etc., you can hear an intriguing "phasing" of their songs because of their differing pulse rates. And the more insects, etc., the more phasing, and therefore the more complexity and seeming randomness in the texture. Similarly with the rhythms of water in a stream or at the beach.

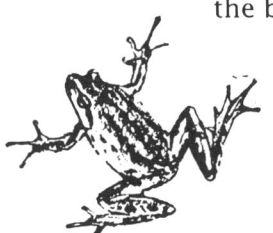 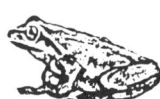 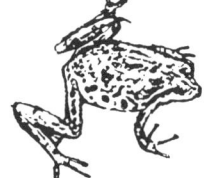 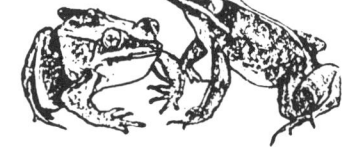

Activity Sequence: Random Pulse 1

1. Get everyone to find a space by themselves and then jump up and down—each in their own time and at their own speed—making a short vocal sound (whoop, ha, hey, etc.) each time their feet touch the ground.

- Get everyone to close their eyes while jumping and listen to the group result.

- As long as each person is trying to discover his natural and comfortable "jump rate" and not trying to follow any group pulse, a natural spectrum of overlapping pulse rhythms will result, i.e., a random rhythmic texture of sounds.

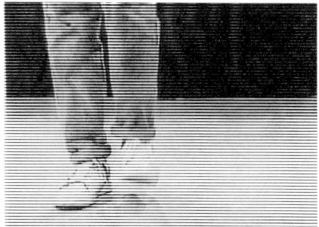

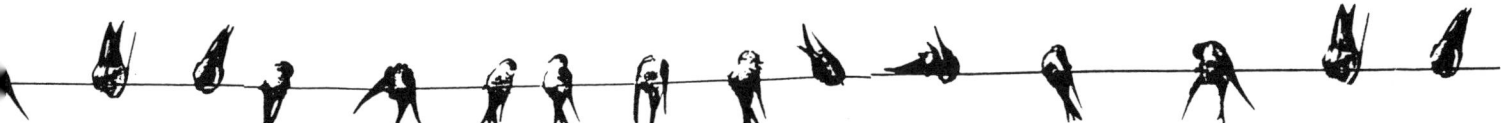

2. Get everyone to choose either a low, medium, or high vocal sound—it'll sound more interesting. Try this in the form of a simple piece made up of progressive entries. That is, one of the group begins jumping and others follow soon after until the whole group is jumping and vocalizing. Everyone then stops in his own time.

    This is a good way to demonstrate how simple, individual parts add together to make a random and complex whole.

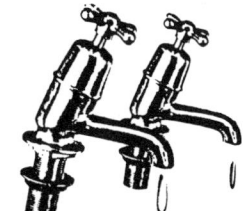

- If the group is quite large, divide it into two, and get one group to jump while the other listens. When the first group starts tailing out, the second group can start in the same manner, one after another.

Points to note and/or discuss

- Any observations of nature relating to seemingly organized and seemingly random.
- The jumping action should be quite relaxed. Let the legs do most of the work and if jumping's hard, try shifting the weight from foot to foot, much like jogging on the spot.

Activity Sequence: Random Pulse 2

1. After doing something energetic (e.g., the previous exercise!) get everyone to monitor their own pulse with eyes closed, and make a short sound (a whistle or vocal "yip") with each pulse beat. Or, pair off and monitor each other's pulse, and make a short sound on each of the other person's pulse beats.

2. Try this first, sounding every beat, then every second beat, then fourth, then eighth, then back through every fourth, second, and then single beats, each person moving through the sequence at his own speed. The sound texture of this piece will gradually move from dense to sparse and back to dense again.

3. One way of arranging this is to have the group stand in a tight circle, with each person putting his ear against the back of the person in front of him.

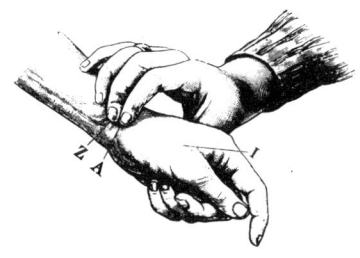

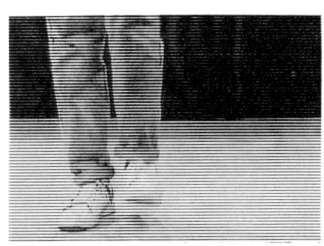

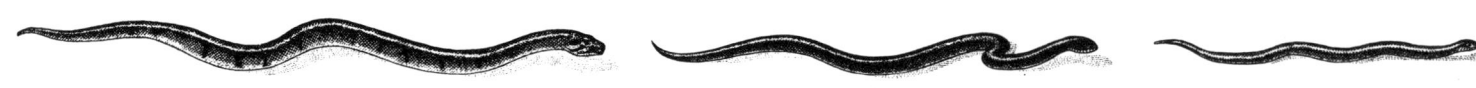

7 ODDS AND EVENS

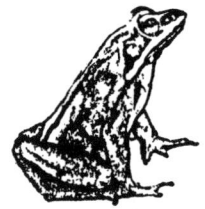

Background

This exercise introduces the idea of rhythmic cycles of different lengths played together to form one longer cycle.

When a group of friends are walking along together, everyone tends to step at a different speed, but from time to time the group will make a single unison footstep. Similarly, but on a much larger scale, the earth, moon, and sun every so often line up to produce a solar eclipse—a dramatic illustration of different cycles briefly coming into synch!

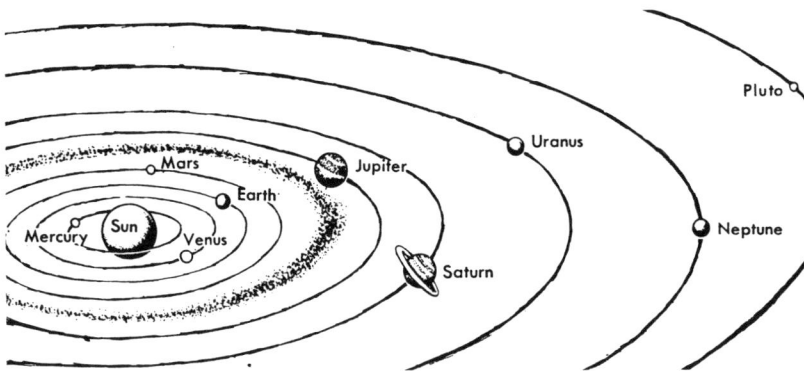

Activity Sequence

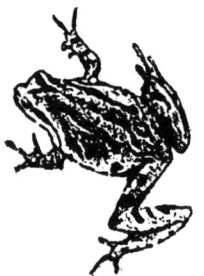

1. Get the group walking in a circle, in step. Let the pace speed up slightly into a relaxed jog, then stop the group, but have them continue to jog on the spot, facing in to the center. The feet barely need to lift off the ground. The movement should be no more than the relaxed transfer of weight from one foot to the other.

2. Split the circle in half to make two lines facing each other, with everyone still jogging in place.

3. With the whole group, practice accenting the footsteps in threes, with a vocal "hey," a clap, and a slightly heavier stamp on the 1 of each cycle of three beats. As in *Walking in a Circle,* you will notice how the accents alternate between right and left because of the odd number.

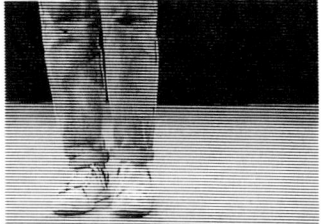

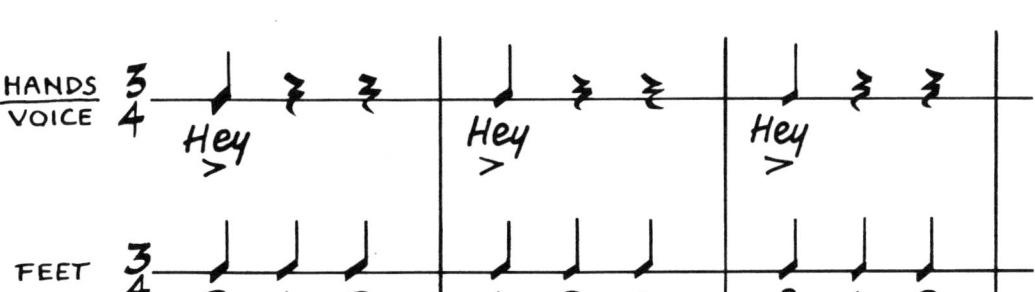

4. When everyone is comfortable with step 3, stop them and get them going with accents on a 4-beat cycle—this time using a vocal "ha" and a clap on the downbeat of each cycle.

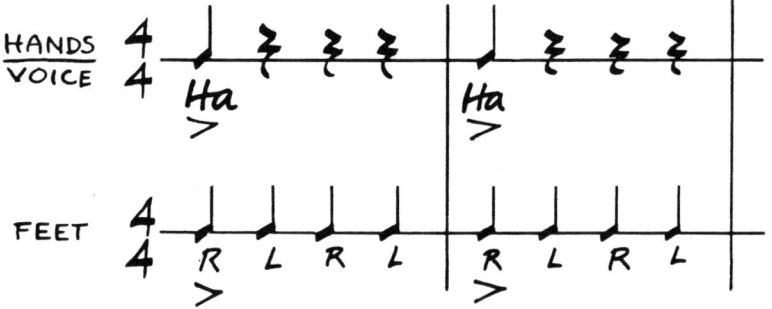

5. When this is going well, make one line the 3s and the other 4s. Start both groups together, ensuring that they keep to the same pulse. Notice that every three 4s and every four 3s, the stamps and vocal sounds fall together. This is the downbeat of the new, long cycle (12) that results from combining the two short ones (3 x 4 and 4 x 3).

6. Sit half the 3s and half the 4s down so that they can listen and watch while the others perform. Then swap over. The effect of the combined cycles is easier to observe when people are not busy counting.

7. Get everyone standing up and start the two groups together again, this

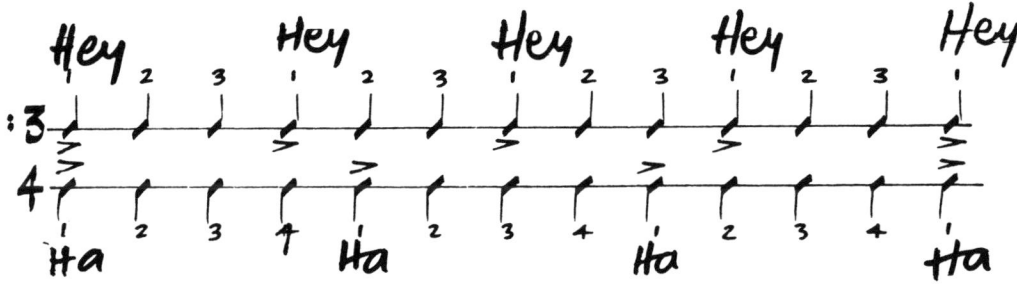

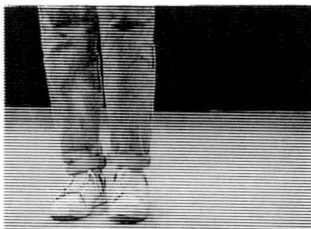

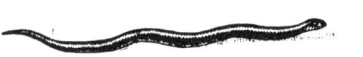
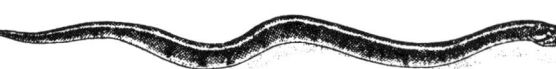

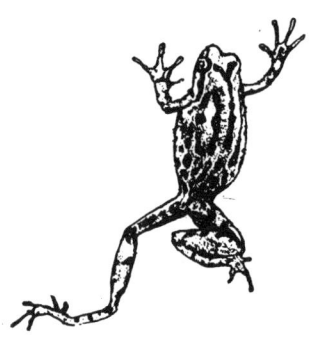

7. Get everyone standing up and start the two groups together again, this time with everyone loudly accenting the point when both groups coincide. (Note: Use the "*One* two three, *two* two three, *three* two three...etc." counting method.) Each time the "big" downbeat comes around, have the groups swap roles (i.e., the 3s become 4s and vice versa.)

8. Now make the 3s advance, while the 4s retreat. This should mean that the two lines push each other back and forth across the room, changing direction every 12 beats.

9. Now try the same whole exercise using 4s against 5s. Use a vocal "ho" sound for the downbeat of the 5s.

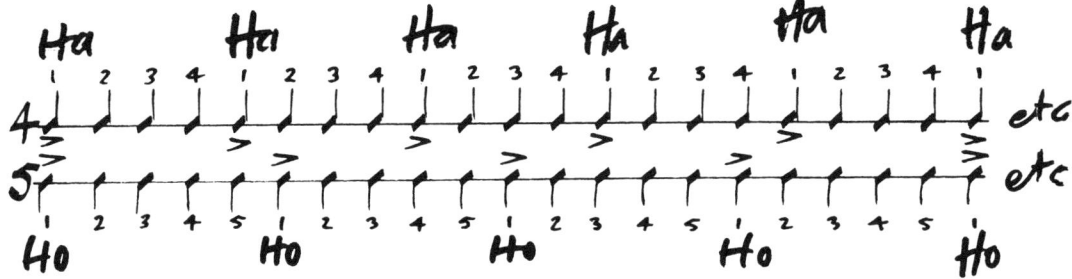

(Again, split the groups in half so they can watch and listen to the effect.)

10. Next, split the class into three groups, in a triangle, facing in to the center. Make one group the 3s, one the 4s, and one the 5s. Start everyone together and see what happens.

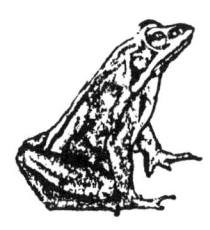
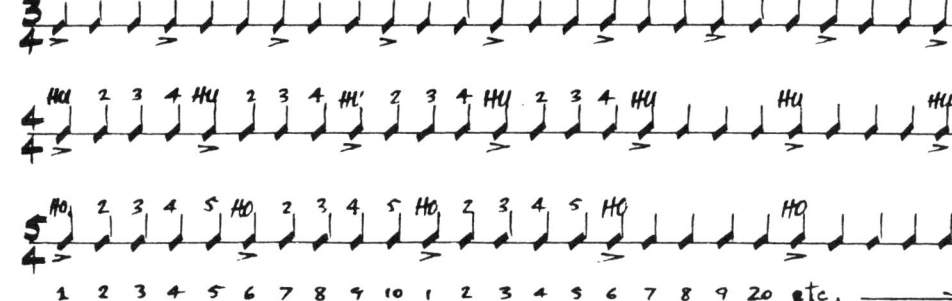

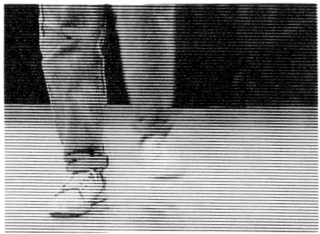
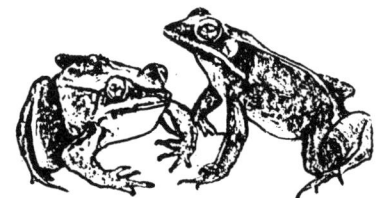
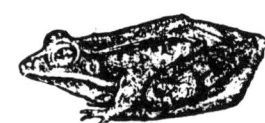

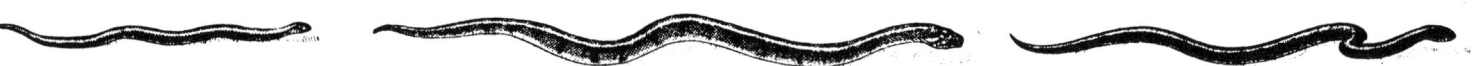

The overall cycle of the *three* subgroups (3s, 4s, and 5s) comes to 60 beats (3 x 4 x 5 = 60). Practice this until everyone knows when the *really big* downbeat is coming.

Note: For the 3s, it will come after 5 lots of *4 x 3*
For the 4s, it will come after 3 lots of *5 x 4*
For the 5s, it will come after 4 lots of *3 x 5*

Developments

Try this last part of the exercise with 3 different consecutive numbers, such as 5, 6, and 7. Try encouraging the group to develop a different foot pattern for each number cycle (keep them simple).

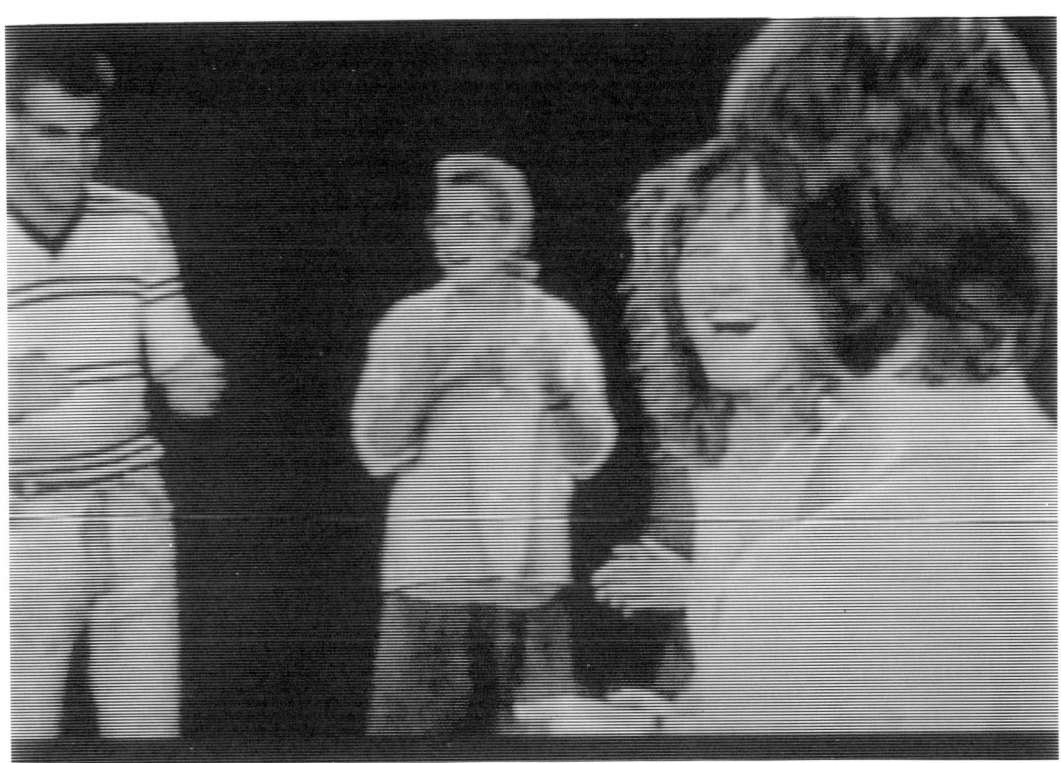

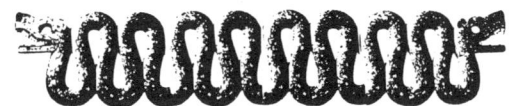

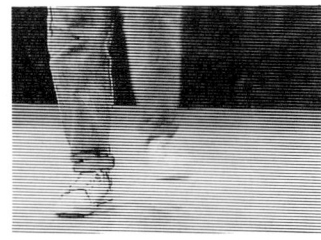

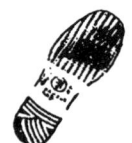
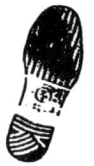
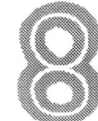

8 STAMPING 1

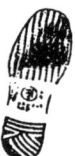
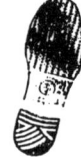
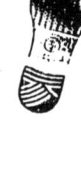
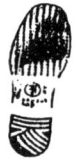
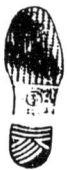

Background

Like *Odds and Evens*, this exercise works with the idea of different-length cycles over a common pulse—only this time, the rhythms are based on a new stamping pattern. This exercise aims to continue developing the skill of holding one rhythmic part against many others.

Activity Sequence

1. First, concentrate on the "stamping" step. Imagine tamping down earth around a tree you've just planted. Your right foot does most of the work, coming flat down on the floor on every on-beat. On each off-beat, lift your weight onto the ball of your left foot.

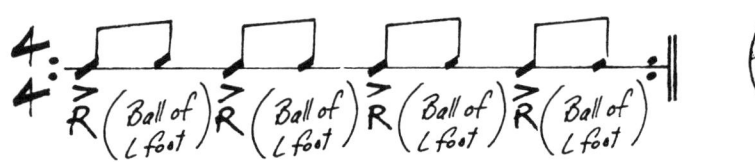
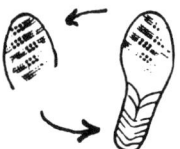

Your legs should be slightly bent and your back straight. Your arms should feel free to swing forward and back once you've got the hang of it.

2. Divide the group into four. Give each group a number (4, 5, 6, or 7), which will be that group's cycle length.

3. Work with each group separately first. Group members should count quietly with each right foot stamp, but shout "1" and clap on the first beat in their cycle. For example, the 4s will go:

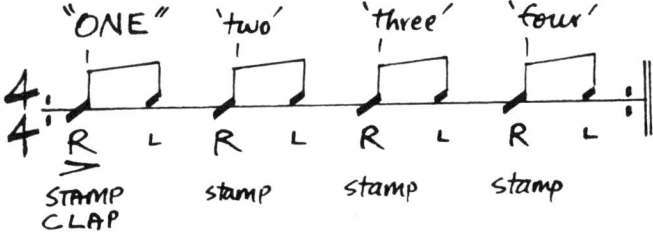

The 5s do the same, but in 5/4, the 6s in 6/4, and the 7s in 7/4.

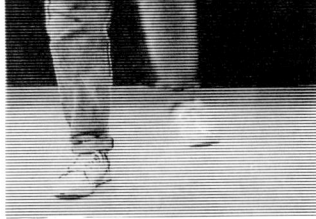

4. Now station the four groups in the four corners of the room. Start the groups off one by one, ensuring that everyone's working to the same pulse. If one group loses the count or pulse, they can just start up again by mutual agreement. It's the *effect* of the interlocking parts that is important in this exercise, rather than the mathematical relationship between them. As long as everyone's feet are on the same pulse, and each group holds on to its cycle, the shouts and claps will form unpredictable but rhythmic accents over the steady beat of the stamp.

5. Now try changing the shouted accents to a range of other sounds. For example, the 7s could make their highest vocal sound, the 6s their lowest, the 5s could whistle, and the 4s could go "sh." (It's good at this point to ask each group to come up with its own sound.) This time you should be able to start all the groups together.

6. As in the previous exercise, split each of the groups in half and separate them, so that you have four groups on one side of the room, and four groups on the other. Start one half of the room off doing the four different cycles together, while the other half watches, listens, and keeps the stamping pattern going.

   After a time, give a signal for the groups on the "listening" side of the room to take over the clap/shout accents from their opposite numbers. Once each "new" group is under way, the "old" group can stop clapping and shouting their accents and start listening (while continuing to mark time with the stamp).

   With a bit of practice you can achieve a seamless transition between performing and listening. It's particularly important to be able to split this exercise up in this way, as the effect of the cycles converging and diverging is difficult to see and hear when you're busy counting your own part.

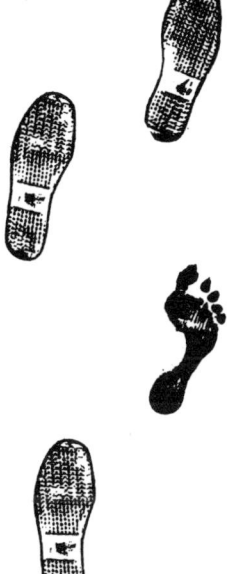

Points to note and/or discuss

If you have three parts with cycles of 4, 5, and 6, and you add a fourth part with a cycle of 7, the complexity and unpredictability of the resulting pattern increases hugely, as does the length of time before the whole cycle begins again. It is the *combination* of differing cycles that creates the forward momentum toward that point where everyone will clap/shout together, just as in the last exercise patterns of 3, 4, and 5 gave rise to a long pattern of 60.

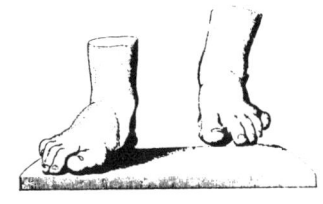

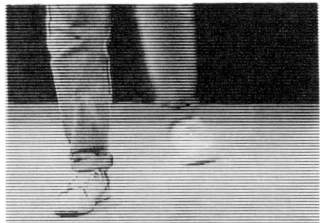

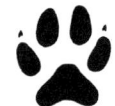
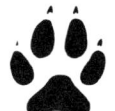

⑨ STAMPING 2

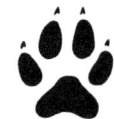
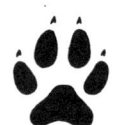

Background

Like some of the longer exercises in this book, this shows how a simple exercise such as *Stamping 1* can be added to and turned into a piece.

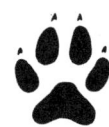

Activity Sequence

1. Divide the group into four subgroups and get each group to stand in one of the four corners of the room, facing into the center of the room.

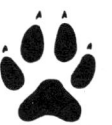

2. As in *Stamping 1,* give each group a number (4, 5, 6, or 7) that will be that group's cycle length. Larger numbers can be good also, but they should be consecutive for best effect.

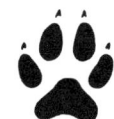

3. Start each group stamping out its cycle—counting quietly on each right foot, and shouting, clapping, and stamping heavily on each downbeat.

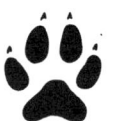

4. When all groups are working well over the common pulse, get each group to edge forward slightly on every *second* one of their cycles. The effect of this will be a gradual converging on the center of the room.

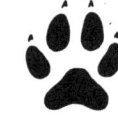

5. When each group reaches the center of the room, each *individual* begins to rotate slowly, at the same time gradually heading out toward the walls again, in any direction. The stamp should become lighter, but still rhythmic. The shout that has been marking the downbeat of each cycle now should become a sung note (each person can pick their own note) for the full length of the cycle. Everyone must now use their eyes and ears to stay in synch with their group—even though by now they will be scattered around the room.

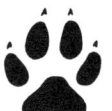

6. From now on, performers should continue to head out toward the wall (turning slowly and singing) or in toward the center of the room (clapping and stamping) at their own individual speed (while still hanging onto their own group's downbeat). Some group members will be heading in while others from the same group are going out.

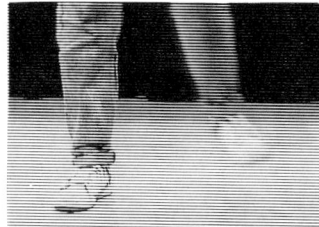

7. To finish, each person should stop singing and stand still when they have touched the wall three times. That means that the closing stages of the piece will be a gradually thinning texture of long sung notes, and the ending will see the whole group standing around the walls.

Note

As in the other stamping exercises, it is very important that everyone holds on to the common pulse that's provided by the stamping pattern.

Development

Once the whole group is confident, try doing the piece with eyes closed (hands out to avoid banging into people), holding onto both pulse and group cycle purely by listening.

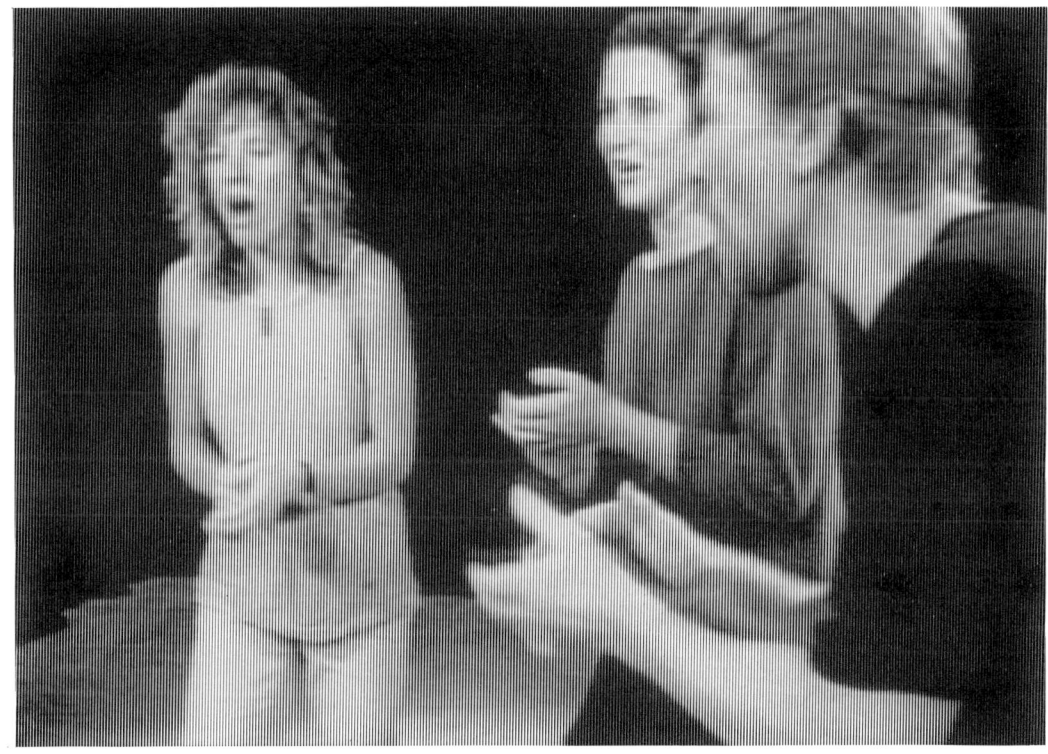

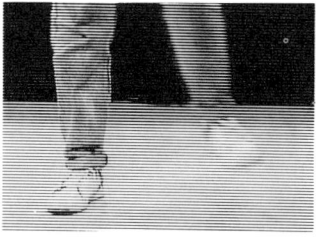

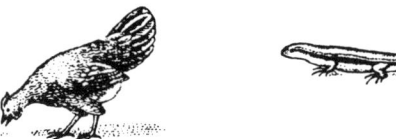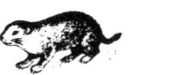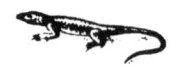

10 OSTINATOS AND SOLOS

Background

This exercise introduces simple, repetitive, rhythmic, and melodic patterns, often referred to as "ostinatos." In this exercise everyone gets to shift around so that the ostinato and "improvised solo" roles are regularly changing.

Activity Sequence

1. Make a large circle and establish the side-to-side foot stamp, counting a 4-beat cycle in unison with the footstepping pattern.

   - Number off around the circle in sets of fours: 1, 2, 3, 4; 1, 2, 3, 4; etc.

   - The first four people each sing a short note (on "ah" or "hah") on thEir number in the 4-beat cycle. Each individual picks his own pitch and sticks to it, so that a repeating 4-note melodic pattern is established—an ostinato.

   Then the next four add their pitches one by one to the first four, 5 in unison with 1, 6 with 2, and so on. At this stage, consideration must be given to how things sound. The notes should combine together, but don't worry about a little dissonance. The sounds will blend and even out as the layering progresses.

   As more cycles are added, each singer has the option of either sticking to his short note or varying the length of the note from 1 to 4 beats long. The volume can also be varied from repeat to repeat. Again, consideration of the overall sound texture is important here.

   This initial stage of layering 4-note melodies over one another continues until everyone in the circle is singing, and don't worry if the last set does not make up a complete 4-beat cycle.

2. When everyone has done this successfully, stop the singing, keep the footstepping going, and explain the next stage. Once everyone is singing, one person from each group, in their own time, can drop out and move in be-

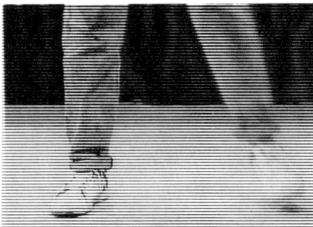

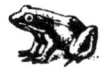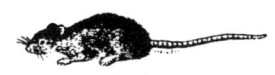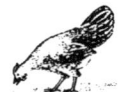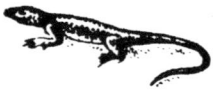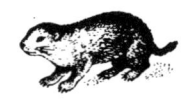

hind any other singer of their choice, take over that singer's pitch and the foot pattern (transposing the pitch up or down an octave where necessary), and then "displace" him with a gentle push. The displaced singer then stops singing and leaves his position, crossing the circle to move in behind someone copying *his* note and movement, and displacing him, and so on.

- To end, a displaced singer has the option of filling the gap left in a 4-beat cycle (and in the circle) instead of displacing another singer. Once this option is taken by one singer, others follow suit until everyone is back in the full circle, after which a signal to finish can be given.

Developments

1. This version follows the same basic format except that it includes an improvisation solo role. Once the initial stage of layering the 4-note melodies is established, up to four singers (each from different ostinato groups) can vacate their places to solo (vocally, with or without body percussion) in center circle before moving across the circle and in behind another singer to displace him. Each singer displaced must solo before displacing another. There should be no more than four soloists at any one time.

   - An alternative ending might be that the soloists (after a goodperiod of role exchanging) displace other singers but they themselves drop out and move around the circle silencing whoever they wish with a tap on the shoulder.

2. Try this with everyone blowing bottles, panpipe style. Collect a wide range of different-size bottles and partially fill them with water. Hold a bottle in one hand and some kind of container in the other hand to pour water off into, so that the pitches can be changed for variation. (*Note:* In this case, it's only necessary to be in *rhythmic* unison with the person you're displacing—don't worry about the pitches).

   A simple structure could be to start with nearly full bottles and gradually empty them—ending the piece when either all the bottles are empty or all the containers are full. The pitches will be somewhat random, but will gradually change from high to low through the course of the piece.

Points to note and/or discuss

- The first singers (or players) to drop out of the 4-note ostinati leave a gap in each cycle. One of the 4 beats in each pattern is now a rest. Those remaining should be careful not to lose the sense of the rest in each pattern.

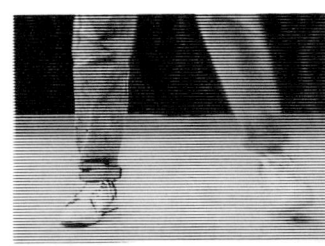

- Soloists should aim to relate their solos to both the 4-beat cycle and to the harmonic bed of ostinati (beware of mindless raving!).
- Alternative ways of ending, such as imposing a time limit.

Advanced exercises

- Try using a 6- or 8-beat cycle. Change the foot-stepping pattern to fit the cycle. For example, if you try 6, use a foot-stepping pattern based on 3 (such as a waltz step on the spot). As skills develop, try a 5 or 7.
- Try this exercise with portable wind and string instruments.

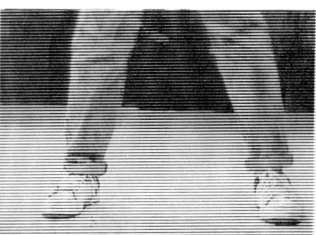

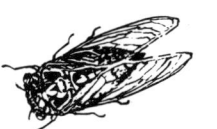
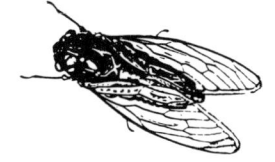

11 PULSE AND IMPROVISATION 1

Background

This is a useful way of introducing a group of nonmusicians to the idea of making a piece of music collectively from simple building blocks.

Activity Sequence

1. Get everyone to sit on the floor in a circle. Start a pulse by tapping on the floor with both palms (an easy tempo of about ♩ = 120 works well). Get everyone doing this in unison.

2. Now get the group to put an accent on the 1 of an 8-beat cycle. While they are getting used to this, explain that everyone must now choose a point in the 8-beat cycle where they are each going to put their solo sound (a sung note, clap, whistle, shout, etc.—one beat or less in length).

3. Moving anti-clockwise around the circle, get each person to introduce their solo sound. People should pick sounds that can be repeated easily every time their chosen beat (or half-beat) in the cycle comes around, and should aim to avoid beats (or half-beats) that are already occupied. As in *Birthday Piece 2*, allow a few repetitions of each new solo sound before the next person in the circle adds hers. Also make sure that the people left playing the "pulse" stay accurate so that the soloists have something to pin their counting on.

4. When all are making their soloing sounds, (and no one's left tapping out the pulse), ask everyone to shut their eyes and listen to the complex, repeating, 8-beat phrase that the group is making.

5. Try changes in dynamics (e.g., "OK, now gradually get softer without losing your part.").

6. Now, still moving anti-clockwise around the circle, get each soloist in turn to return to tapping the pulse. Again, leave several repetitions between

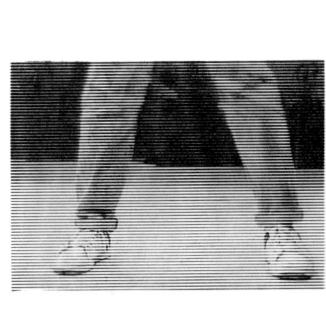

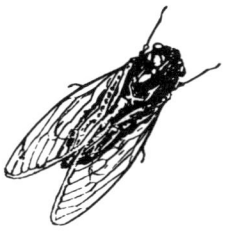

soloists dropping out, to allow each subtle change in texture to establish itself. When all are back on the pulse, get the whole group to play the 8-beat cycle through eight times, getting softer and softer, and stopping on the last count of 8.

With a little practice, it should be possible for the group to perform the whole piece without prompting. You can do it several times in succession without anyone's getting bored, as each time they can choose both a new sound and a new place to put it.

7. Make up, or have someone in the group suggest, an 8-beat rhythm phrase that the whole group can clap in unison. For example:

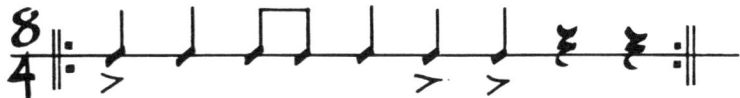

Use this as a sort of refrain between the longer, evolving sections. This can be signalled by a count in from the group leader.

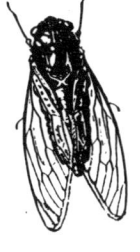

8. If a blackboard is available, write a flow diagram of the piece on it. For example:

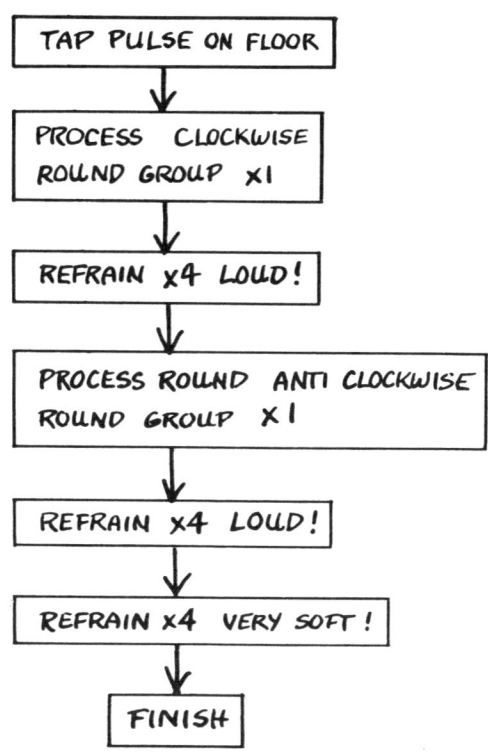

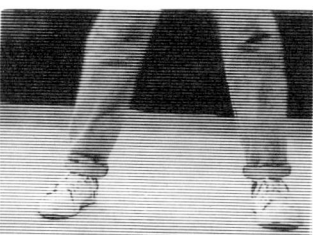

30

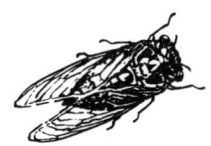
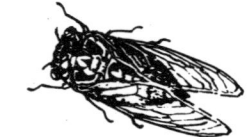

Perform this version of the piece. Now ask members of the group to think up other possible flow diagrams, and get the group to perform these. This can be a good jumping-off point for discussions about structure and composition.

Developments

1. Try the exercise with hand-held instruments (clavés, cymbals, wood blocks, drums, etc.). If melodic instruments are included, it is best to agree on a key (e.g., C pentatonic, E-minor, etc.). When the melodic instruments are playing the pulse, they could be combining to sound a chord on every beat. You can also slightly expand the solos to phrases that are 2 or 3 beats long. This can make it more interesting.

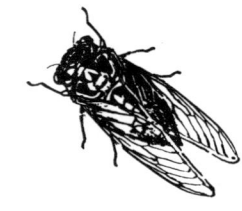

2. Try this same 8-beat exercise with a text, for example a page of a newspaper, as the "sound material." The pulse people each choose one word and repeat it on the beat, while the soloists say short phrases, chosen at random from the newspaper—varying the tone and emphasis. The refrain can be a whole headline spoken in unison by the entire group. Once everyone gets confident with this, gestures can be added to the phrases.

3. Try all of these options using different cycle lengths.

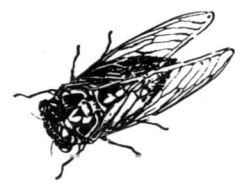

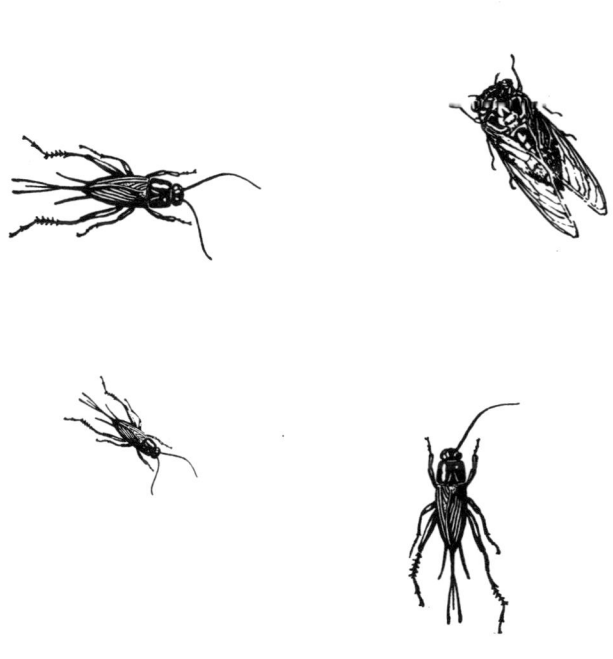

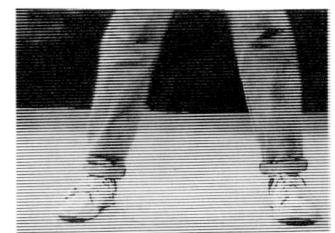

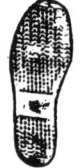
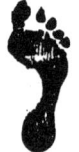

12 ONS AND OFFS 1

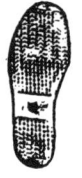
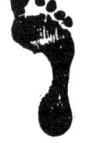

Background

Rhythms that combine on-beats and off-beats make music lively and interesting. The worlds great rhythm traditions—Indian, African, Indonesian, and Afro-Cuban—have developed on-beat, off-beat patterning into sophisticated languages. In this exercise off-beats are treated in a way that makes them as natural to play as on-beats.

Activity Sequence

1. Divide the group into two groups facing each other and begin the side-to-side foot-stamp pattern at around ♩ = 120. Starting on the right foot, count in and clap the following on/off cycle at the same speed as the footstamp.

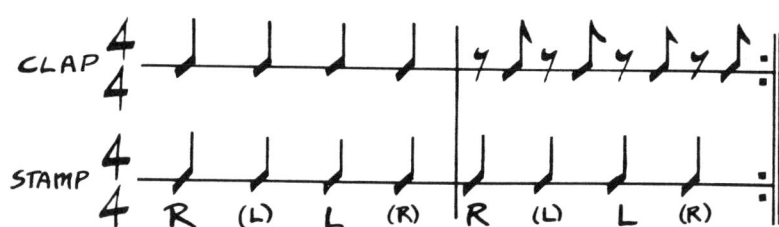

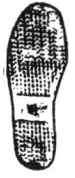
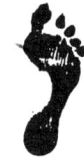

- This is the basic cycle—one bar of on-beats, one bar of off-beats. The off-beats should not feel any different from the on-beats. They are the same distance apart in time and are played with the same two hands.

- Use your feet to tell you where both on-beats and off-beats should fall—the on-beats in unison, and off-beats in the middle, exactly halfway between—and stay relaxed; they'll come right.

2. Next, explain how one group "goes out" by adding in one extra bar of on-beats ahead of playing the next cycle. In other words, the on-beat half of the cycle is repeated, once only.

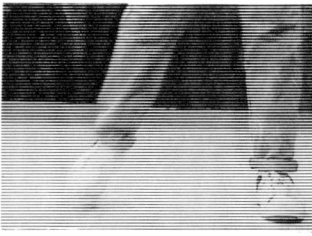

32

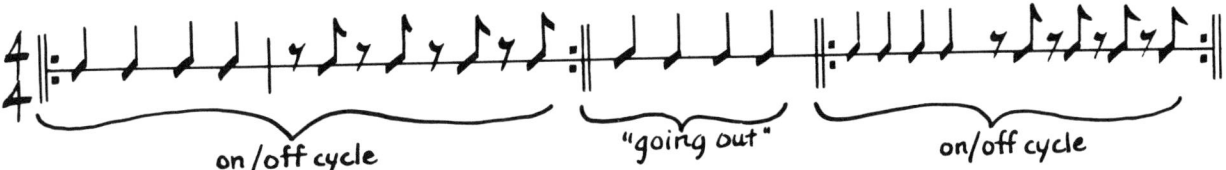

- This single addition puts the two groups into opposition. A "hocket"-type relationship is made where the combined effect of the two groups is one of regular quavers. For example:

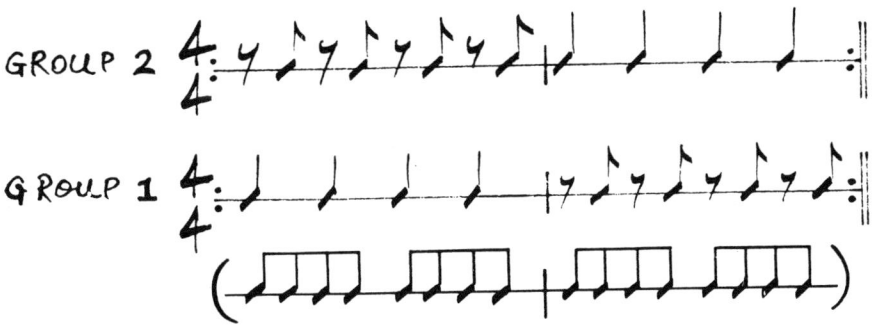

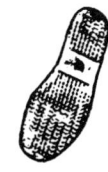

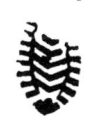

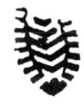

- Try this starting off the pattern in unison, and then each group taking turns to go out and return to unison. Use eye contact within the group to signal when to go out, or appoint a leader to cue changes.

3. Now get everyone into a large circle and divide the circle into three sub-groups. Start the groups in unison doing the foot-stepping pattern and the basic on/off cycle. Group 1 goes out first, followed by group 2, to join group 1. Lastly, group 3 goes out and everybody should be back in unison ready to start another cycle. Continue with each group independently cueing changes, and call a halt at a point when everyone is back in unison.

4. Try all these over a half-speed foot pulse. It involves a lot less foot work and will make the performing much more relaxed. (If the group is experienced enough, you could try this from the outset.)

Developments

1. Try doing the same thing in 3/4, using a cycle of 3 on-beats and 3 off-beats. Start first with everyone in unison, and then try the same procedure as described in steps 2 and 3 above. Then try cycles of 5 and 6.

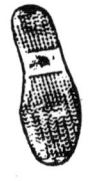

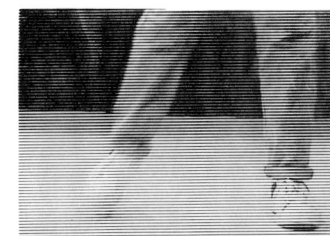

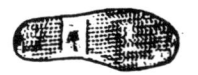
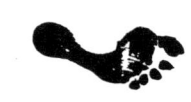
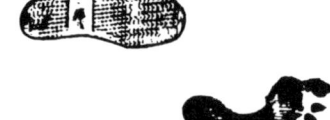
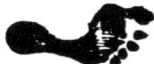

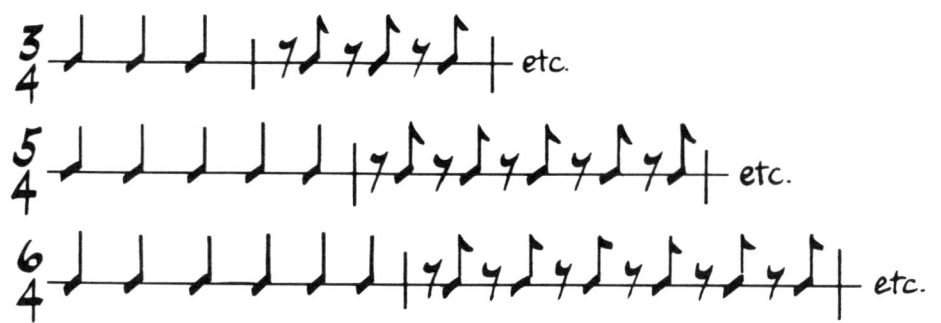

- With these variations and the basic cycle, counting the on-beats through both halves of a cycle will help everyone keep track of the "form," (also a useful skill for everyone to learn individually).

2. Adding vocals
   (a) try adding bar-long voice chords, as illustrated next, to the first notes of each bar in the on/off cycle.

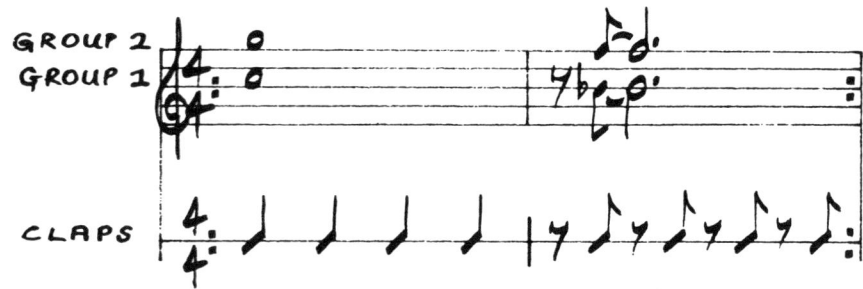

- The interval between the chords is one whole tone. Demonstrate this for each of the groups by singing or playing each note sequence, and then get them to try it together.

- Here are three more vocal variations to try with the on/off clapping.

(b) shorter sung notes in unison with the claps.

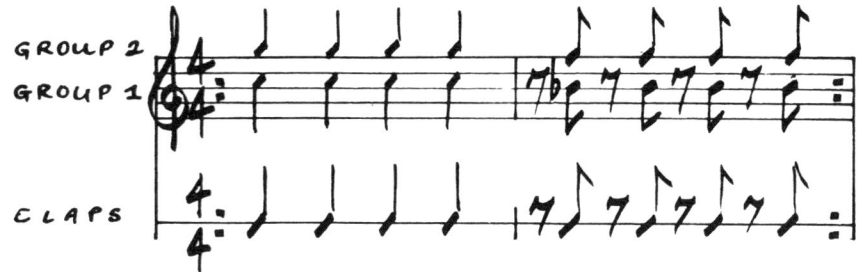

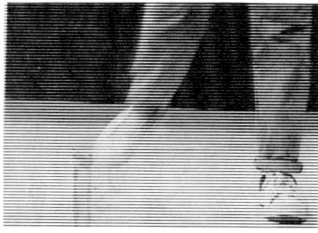

(c) and (d) combinations of the two.

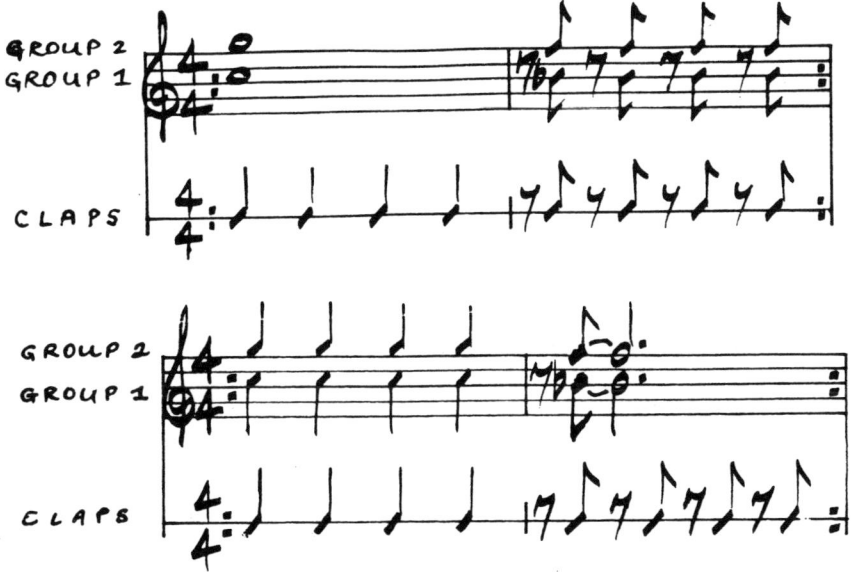

Demonstrate these four variations by first singing each one with the whole group together, and then get one group to go out against the other on each one. (When you repeat the first bar to go out, repeat the pitch of that bar as well.)

- Adding vocals takes a bit of time, so don't despair. You may find it helpful to get the whole group doing some simple chord singing as a warm-up first (see Appendix 2).

- Get the group individually ad-libbing pitches from this common starting point. It increases the interest straight away.

3. Split up into four groups, with two of the groups in 4/4 and two in 3/4. Give each pair of groups two notes to sing. For example:

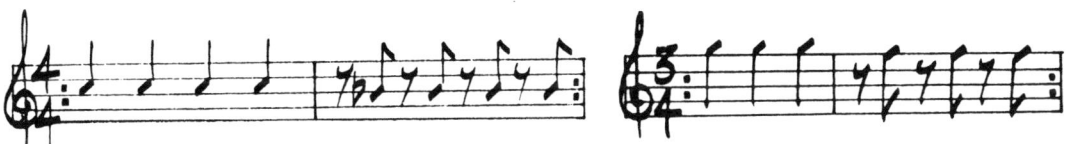

Establish a common pulse with the side-to-side foot stamp, and on a signal, begin the groups clapping their respective cycles, first in unison and then phasing within the pairs.

Next add the vocals, one group after another or each pair together on a signal. To begin with use the notes given out, but after a while, ad-lib pitches and 2-bar rhythm variants as listed earlier in item 2.

- Try the same exercise in 4/4 and 5/4.

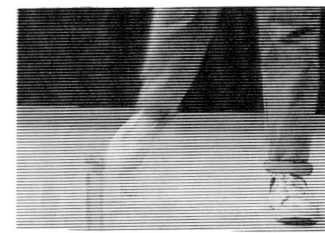

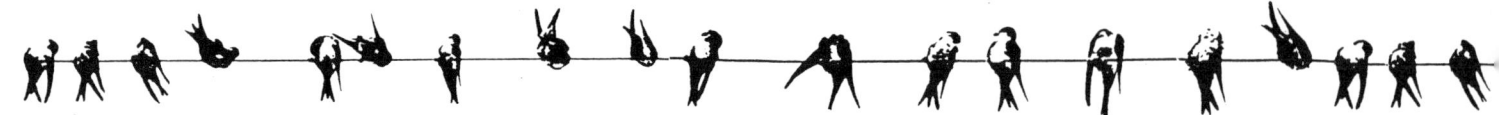

Advanced Exercise

A more structured harmonic result can be achieved by each group's moving their two notes, one scale step at a time, up and down a prearranged scale common to all groups. The overall effect is a shifting harmonic texture of contracting and expanding intervals, but for this to work effectively, each group needs to develop a sense of its being one bit in the chord construction. For detailed discussion on how to develop this step by step, see Appendix 3.

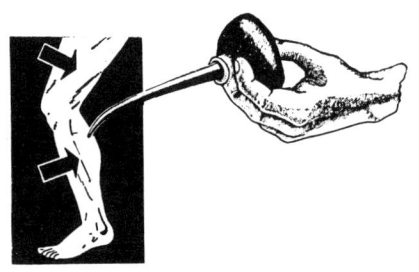

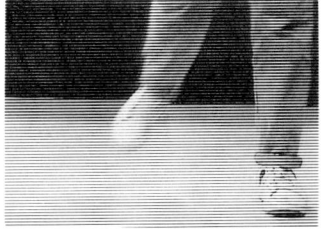

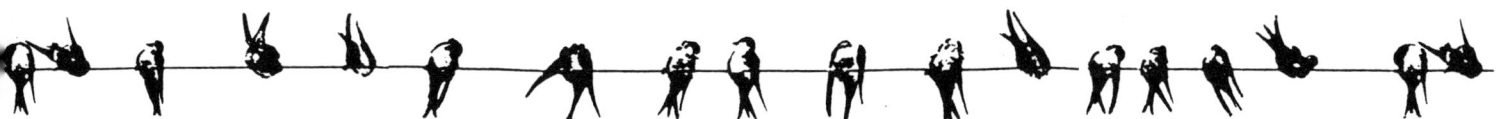

13 ONS AND OFFS 2

Background

Ons and offs 2 combines ideas developed in *Ons and Offs 1* with movement and the substituting of rests for notes. In this piece, give your hands a break from clapping and prepare as many (hand-sized) paired lengths of 1"- to 2"-diameter dowel (or any other suitable wood) as there are players.

Activity Sequence

1. Form four groups, two to perform 4/4 on/off cycles and the other two, cycles in 5/4.

   - Position the four groups in the four corners of the room with pairs opposite each other diagonally and establish vocal pitches for each pair of groups (the same as, or different from, the previous exercise).

   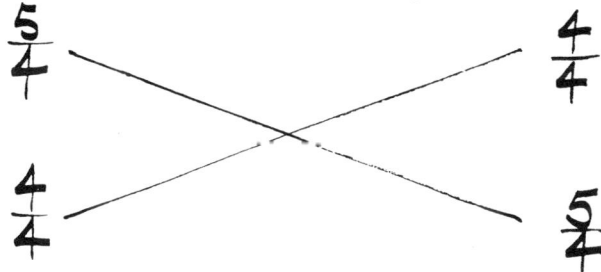

2. Form each group into a circle of its own and count everyone off on a unison footstamp. Get one person in each group to be responsible for keeping the foot pulse in unison with the other groups.

3. On a signal (5 quarter notes sounded on a pair of clavés), the two 5/4 groups start the 5/4 on/off pattern using the clavés, and after two of these cycles the two 4/4 groups begin. Shortly after, the four groups go out within their pairs and start the vocal rhythms.

   - When each group starts to sing, each also starts to move slowly toward the center of the space, maintaining the unison footstamp.

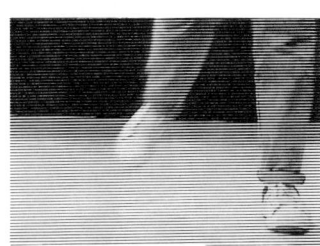

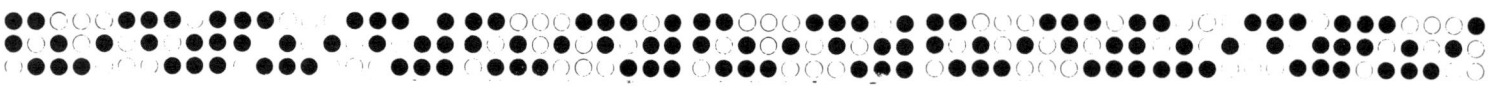

- When the four groups meet, they reform into one large circle and (on a signal) without a break, the two 5/4 groups change their rhythm to 4/4 (or vice versa, the two 4/4 groups change to 5/4) so that everyone is now playing the same cycle (though not necessarily in the same *part* of the cycle).

4. When all four groups are working in the same time signature, individual players can start substituting rests for notes in the percussion rhythms, gradually "devolving" the rhythm texture to nothing, leaving only the singing.

    When each player ends their rhythm playing, they also stop the foot-stamp pattern. The singing should continue for a while and end in unison on a signal.

    Here is an example of how an individual player might substitute rests for notes in her percussion part (while continuing singing).

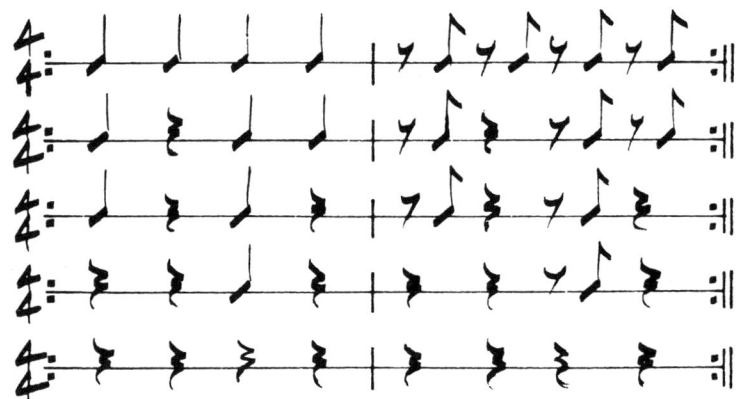

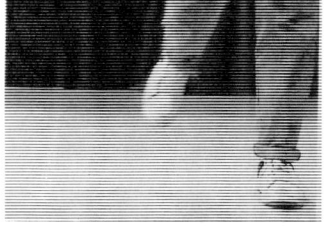

14 ONS AND OFFS 3

Background

The main aim of this game is to get everyone familiar with a wide range of odd- and even-numbered on/off patterns, plus encourage a high degree of focus. The game starts out with clapping and explores a full range of number cycles from 1 to 10, but the principle can be applied to any kind of instrumentation and provides the basis for an interesting sounding piece. It can be practiced alone, and be performed in pairs as well as in larger groups.

This is a great warm-up and focusing exercise before any performance that requires rhythmic accuracy.

Activity Sequence

1. Pair off, or divide the group into subgroups of 4 to 6 people per group, and choose a number cycle between 1 and 10 on which to start. (A cycle of 4 is usually the easiest for getting things started.)

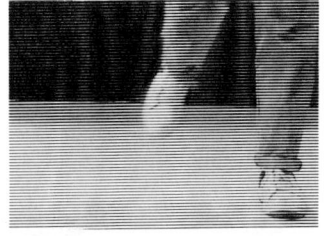

2. Establish the half-speed, side-to-side foot pulse at a relaxed pace, and count in the selected unison on/off cycle.

3. When the unison cycle is established, any individual within a pair or a subgroup may call a change to any other on/off cycle within the 1 to 10 range.

   - The call, and the change that follows, applies only to that particular pair or subgroup.

   - The call must occur at the start of the off-beat half of a cycle so there's plenty of warning to make the change together.

4. After the call is made, the new cycle is established for a bit and then another call is made for another unison change, and so on, until each pair or group has explored the full range of cycles from 1 to 10. Once again, remember that although everyone is on the same foot pulse, each pair or group is working through the range of numbers in its own order, at its own pace.

5. Now try the same thing but with the going-out option included as well. (This requires each group to divide into two—as in *Ons and Offs 1*.)

   - To start, it is useful to get the group back into unison before making the call to change the cycle. As you get more practiced, you can call and make the change while the group is still in the out phase.

Developments

- Try this at different speeds, gradually taking it as fast as possible without sacrificing accuracy. Be careful not to speed up or slow down once the speed is established. Then try incorporating an accelerando or de-accelerando, or both.

- Try this exercise with instruments, including the voice. Players of wind instruments will need to leave out the off half of the cycle in order to make a call. Pitches can be improvised or a harmonic plan can be devised in advance.

- If the group is very advanced, try dropping the foot-stepping pattern.

Points to note and/or discuss

- It's good at the start to count aloud on the beat through both halves of the cycle, and then later just mentally.

- Tension is a barrier to precision. The more relaxed you are, the easier and more precise the on/off cycle will be, also.

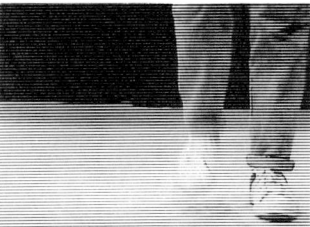

15 PULSE AND IMPROVISATION 2

Background

This exercise is similar to *Pulse and Improvisation 1,* but involves a less rigid structure and a greater degree of improvisation. It requires each player to have a wide range of percussion sound sources.

Find junk and other sound sources that have great sounds and divide them into categories of wood, metal, glass, skin, plastic, etc. Your sound sources should vary in timbre (i.e., tonal quality), in pitch (some high and low), and in the duration of notes (longs and shorts). Everyone should also have some kind of drum (skin or plastic).

- Players in the group each select two or three sound sources to fit each category of low, medium, and high pitch, and arrange them at sitting or standing level—whichever suits your situation.
- A good way to begin arranging the instruments is for each player to sit or kneel at floor level with her instruments placed around her in a semi-circle, in groups of low, medium, and high pitches (arranged low to high, from left to right). The instruments may need suspending or supporting, and there are some simple suggestions for this in Appendix 6.

Activity Sequence

1. Get everyone to arrange into a circle of sorts, so that they are facing inward and can see each other.

    - There is no foot-stamp pulse for this one. Everyone will need to rely on "feel."

2. An elected player begins a slow drum pulse (about ♩ = 80), and one after another, all the players join in, softly, in unison.

3. Players then gradually depart from the pulse in their own time, improvising by adding off-beats and decorations to the pulse.

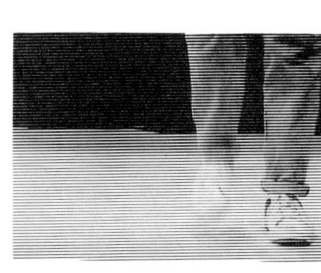

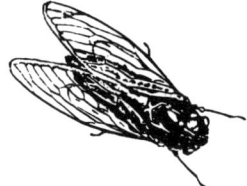

- The pulse must never disappear, and a player can only depart from it if two or more players are keeping it going.
- Everyone alternates between pulse playing and decorating the pulse. Players who lose the pulse must stop, listen, and then resume, first playing the pulse and then later improvising on it.

4. The player who begins is the first to stop. The others follow suit one after another, each in her own time.

   For a warm-up to this, sit in a circle and perform the same piece using body percussion and mouth sounds.

Development

When some percussion-playing skills have developed, collect together a wide range of drums and try a version of this outdoors.

Points to note and/or discuss

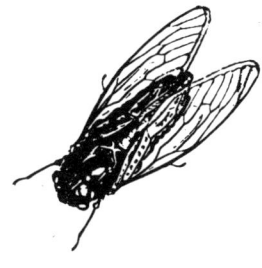

- Discuss the difference between accompaniment playing and solo playing.
- Discuss ways of combining your high, medium, and low sounds into rhythmic patterns and including these rhythms as part of your improvisation. (See Appendix 4.)
- Note how large groups commonly get faster and louder and louder. Keep a solid sense of the pulse, and listen to one another at all times. Be conscious of dynamics and play softly more than loudly.

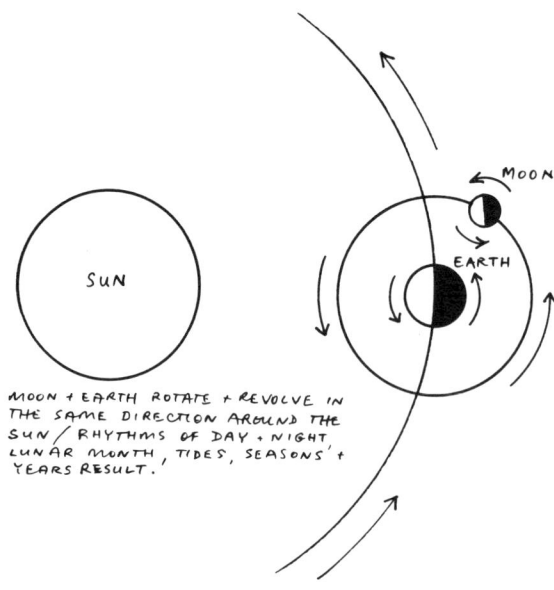

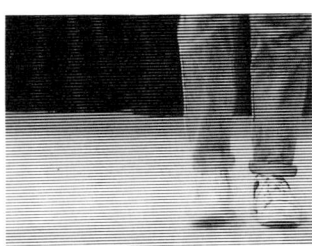

16 ACTION LOOP GAMES

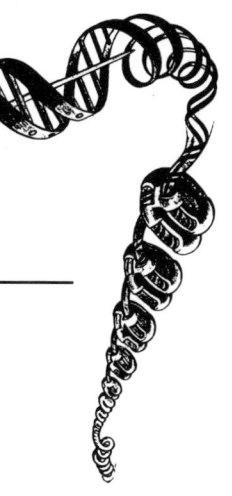

Background

Repetitive actions and gestures are a natural part of most work activities, and these in turn have inspired much traditional and contemporary dance. The first two of these loop games are adaptations of an "improvisation rite" devised by Alvin Curran in 1970 for the London-based "Scratch Orchestra."

These games can create some quite beautiful group gesture-dances—as well as being mostly silent, and therefore a good break among all the clapping and shouting exercises!

It's difficult to do these pieces with more than about eight people, so if your group is large, try:

- Having one group at a time performing them for the others.

- Having two or more groups performing simultaneously.

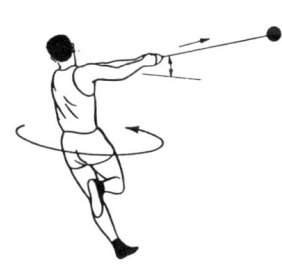

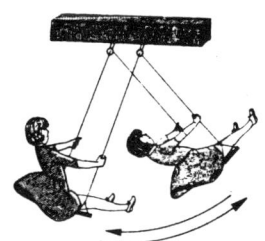

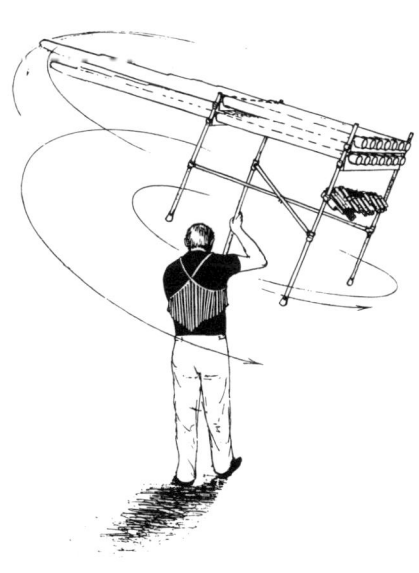

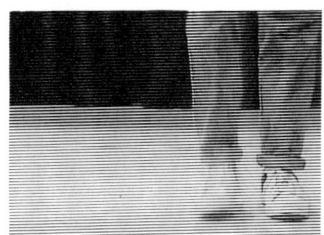

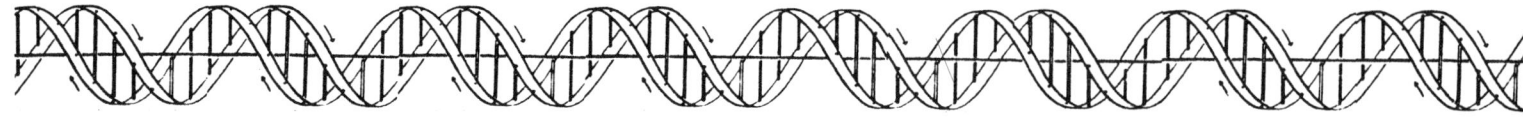

Activity Sequence

1. Get the group to stand in a circle so everyone can see each other. One person begins by making an easily imitated gesture—something really simple that can be easily repeated over and over as an action loop. Everyday gestures and expressions are good. The action should be performed in a relaxed way, with a short pause between each repeat. *Note:* There doesn't need to be any reference to a pulse.

2. Going anti-clockwise, the next person in the circle watches the first action till he feels he can imitate it perfectly. He then does so, adding a simple action of his own on the end of the imitated one. This person then continues to repeat his new, longer, action loop in his own time, again with a short pause between repeats. *Note:* This new loop doesn't have to stay in synch with the first person's.

3. This continues around the circle with the action loop gradually growing until the last person is repeating a movement sequence comprised of all of the group members' gestures.

4. Now, going clockwise from the person doing this "full" movement sequence, each person begins to imitate the complete loop in unison with the last person—until everybody is performing it together. The last one to get into unison can signal "twice more," so that the whole group finishes as one.

Developments

1. Try the same exercise over the side-to-side foot step—this time using short rhythm phrases (made up of hand claps and body slaps) rather than gestures. As in the preceding version, the phrase gets gradually added to as it moves anti-clockwise around the group, and then, moving clockwise, everyone gradually learns the complete phrase. Unlike the previous exercise, though, everyone's phrase (although they're all of different lengths) should have a precise relationship to the pulse. This should make for an exciting and complex rhythm piece, where a single, long unison phrase gradually emerges from a dense, syncopated texture.

2. Still in a circle (or semi-circle if you are performing to an audience), get the group to establish a very slow side-to-side foot step (♩ = 80). One person now makes a gesture 1 beat long. This becomes 1 of a repeating 4-beat cycle.
   After a while, someone else makes his own gesture on one of the empty beats (2, 3, or 4), and repeats it in the same way. One at a time, and in their own time, two more people enter, with the result that, somewhere in the group, there is a gesture on each of the 4 beats. From now on, the rest of the group can, one by one, join in with a gesture that is already established.

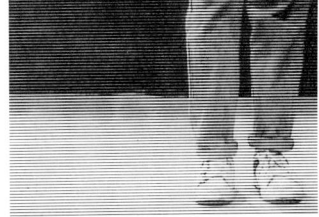

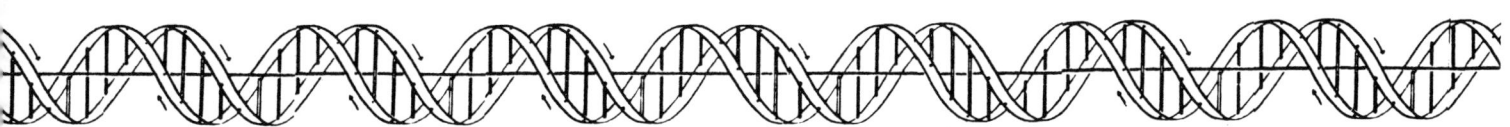

Once everybody is "in," performers begin, one at a time, to incorporate each other's gestures into their own cycle—until eventually everyone is doing the same, slow, 4-beat action loop in unison. Remember that the process is more important than the "destination." Allow a few repetitions' breathing space for each new change to the overall texture.

When everyone has repeated the unison loop several times, one performer adds a fifth gesture, and then continues to repeat this new 5-beat cycle. The others carry on with their old 4-beat cycle another four times (all the while checking up on the nonconformist to see what he is doing); then they all change in unison to the new 5-beat cycle.

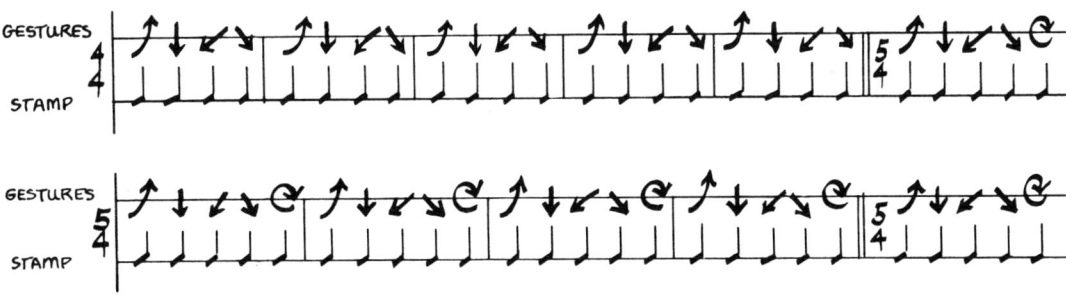

By continuing in the same way, the action loop can be extended to a 7-beat cycle, an 8-beat cycle, or more. (Once the group notices that one member has added an extra gesture to his cycle, the number of extra repetitions the group must play before shifting to that new cycle is always equal to the number of beats of the cycle they're currently on.)

To finish the piece, each person in his own time could begin replacing gestures with stillness, so that everyone has one still beat in their movement phrase, then two still beats, and so on until there are no more gestures.

3. Try exactly the same procedures as in 1 and 2 but with

- vocal sounds, spoken words/phrases, extracts from texts
- combinations of movements and words/vocal sounds
- musical phrases (using voices and/or instruments)

Points to note and/or discuss

To give enough time for the gestures, it's very important that this exercise doesn't speed up. Note that all of these pulsed action loop games can also work well if the pulse is external. The workshop leader can provide the pulse on claves, maracas, etc., or organize the audience (if there is one) to provide a pulse of steady finger clicks.

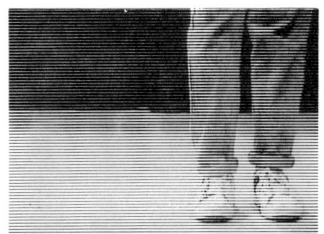

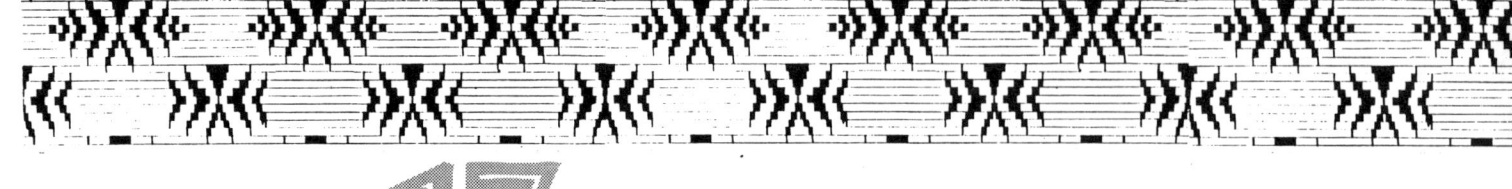

17 COMBINATION 1

Background

In this game, polyrhythmic ideas introduced in *Odds and Evens* and *Stamping 1 and 2* are further developed. Confidence is built with playing in odd- and even-numbered rhythm cycles and with improvising solos over the resulting bed of rhythm. A system of role exchange (first used in *Ostinatos and Solos*) is used to get everyone familiar with the various options. Stage 1 uses all voice and body percussion sounds. Stage 2 adds instruments.

Activity Sequence

Stage 1: Voice and body percussion sounds

1. The foot-step pattern to start is a relaxed jogging action on the spot—much like walking, but with the weight essentially on the balls of the feet.

2. Divide the group into four and give each group a number (3, 4, 5, 6), which will be it's rhythmic cycle length. Any low, consecutive number sequence is fine but 3, 4, 5, 6 is good to begin with. Get each group to count its cycle in time with the foot pulse and clap together on the first beat of the cycle.

3. Get each group to devise a simple foot and body movement pattern suggested by the "feel" of the cycle; for example, the 3s might do a waltz step on the spot and the 4s might do a variation on the side-to-side foot-stepping pattern, and so on, but each one should still be accompanied by a clap on the first beat of the cycle. This establishes an identity for each number cycle. Have the groups demonstrate their pattern one at a time before moving onto 4.

4. Now add a vocal sound to the clap on the 1 of each cycle. Get each group to decide on its own unique sound, which it should be able to alternate between a high and a low pitch.

5. Form a large circle with small gaps between the four groups, and start the groups off in sequence beginning with the 3s as follows: 4 x 3s, then 4s enter; 4 x 4s, then 5s enter; 4 x 5s, then 6s enter.

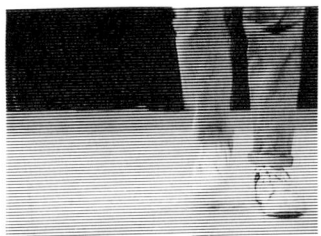

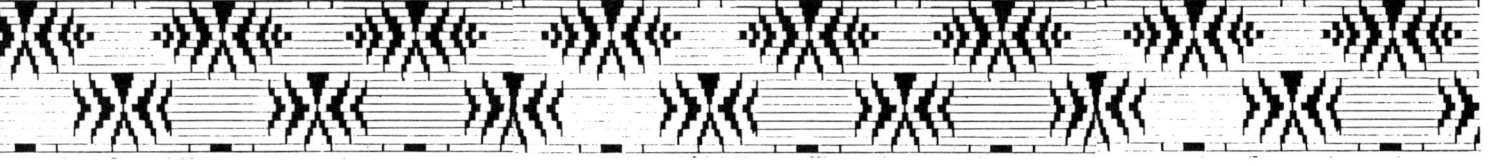

6. Next, get each group to try doubling up the speed of each number cycle (the easiest way to understand this is to think of it as fitting two units into one, i.e., by halving the length of the first cycle). For the even-numbered cycles this is easy, but the odd-numbered ones may need demonstrating as follows:

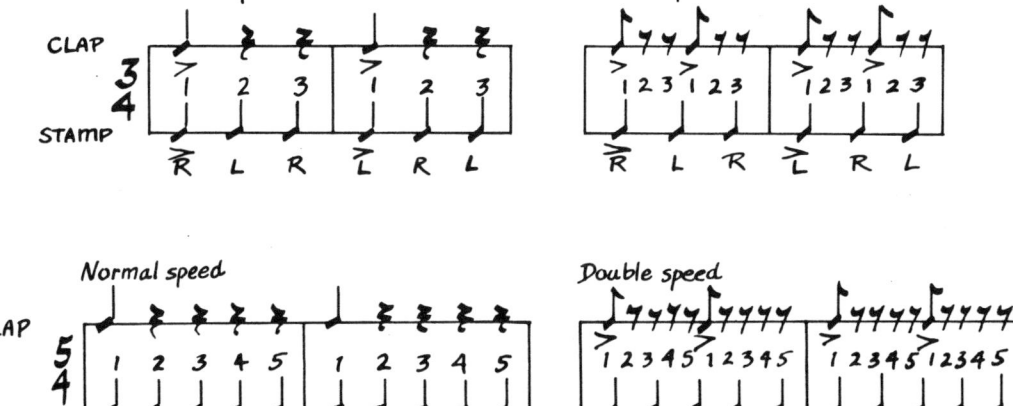

- The foot pulse speed should not change, and high and low pitches should still alternate.

- Try alternating a set number of repeats for each speed, e.g., 8 x 3 (standard speed) and 8 x 3 (double speed)—or have a leader in each group cuing the changes in and out.

- Try the four groups together with standard speed/double-speed alternations.

6. Now explain the role of the soloist/improviser as follows:

- When the number cycles are well established, any one player from each group can leave her place in the group to improvise a solo in center circle.

- Solos should be rhythmic and use a range of vocal and/or body percussion sounds.

- After soloing, the player moves across the circle to join a new group (different to that she has left). This is done by passing across the circle and standing behind a player of her choice, imitating the sound and action relating to the number cycle, and then taking over that role by "displacing" the player with a gentle push (as in *Ostinatos and Solos*). The displaced player should then improvise a solo, and following that, move

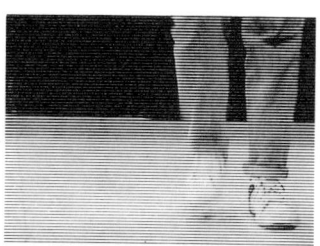

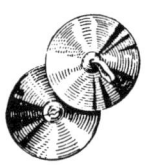

across the circle to join another group by displacing a player as described previously, and so on.

- Solos provide the triggering device for role changes, which, once started, continue until the game ends.

- Note that there can be no more than one soloist from each group at a time.

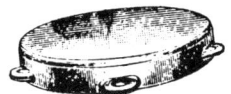

- To end, the leader can simply call things to a halt by stopping one group after another—or after a period of role changing, the soloists can trigger new solo roles and instead of joining a new group, drop out to watch and listen. Each new soloist follows suit, and the groups gradually diminish in size until there are no more soloists.

Stage 2: Adding instruments

1. Collect percussion instruments to match the categories of metal, wood, drum (including skin and tube-percussion), and rattles (including shakers and scrapers).

    Station the four categories of instruments in the space so they are easily accessible from the front and behind (in four corners or in a circular format is good), give each group a number as in stage 1, and agree on a common key or modal reference, e.g., C pentatonic or D Dorian, etc. (see Appendix 1).

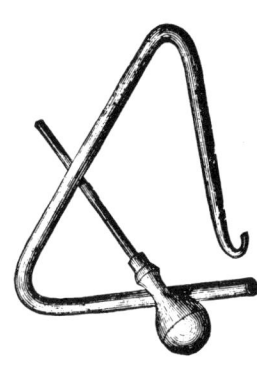

- Instruments can be at floor level or on tables, as appropriate (but if they are hand-held, a foot-step and movement pattern is still possible).

- Some instruments inhibit physical movement and a conducting role may be necessary, in which case, one person with shakers can be assigned to a pulse-keeping role.

- Let each group decide on high/low pitch alternations, and make suggestions where necessary. Get the groups to independently rehearse their rhythm cycles, as in stage 1, and then try all the groups together with either a unison start or staggered entries, as in stage 1.

2. Next add the improv/solo role. Each soloist can perform on a hand-held percussion instrument, or with voice and body percussion, or the two in combination. If the solo is on an instrument, the instrument must be returned to its station when the player moves off to join another group.

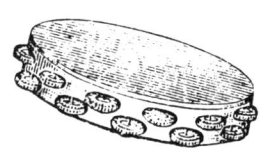

- Follow the same procedures for beginning and ending the piece that are outlined in stage 1.

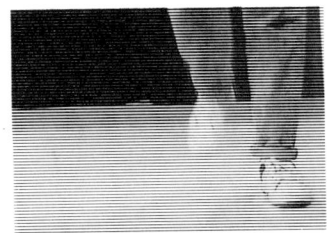

Developments

- Try different number combinations with the various versions of this game; for example, 4, 5, 6, 7; 5, 6, 7, 8; 3, 5, 7, 9; etc.

- Devise rhythmic phrases to fit the number cycles. These phrases can be cued in by a signal and played as unison "refrains" within the groups (in a similar way to the refrains in *Pulse and Improvisation 1*).

- Try portable solo instruments, other than percussion, that can be carried from place to place and used when needed.

Things to note and discuss

- The importance of group volume and dynamics and the relationship of the group sound to the soloist.

- Solos give the opportunity to express musicianship. Try making a solo relate to the feel of the number group you have just left. If any in the group have reservations about soloing, encourage them to use the on/off patterns introduced in *Ons and Offs 3*. These patterns can be directly related to the number cycles of the different groups and can form a good basis for improvisations.

- The conductor's role need not be limited to one person and one sound source. Role exchanges can occur by the conductor's nominating someone else to take her place.

- Instruments at your disposal should conform to clear timbral distinctions, e.g., wood, metal, membranes, and shakers, so that each group has a clear sound identity. If this is not possible, it is better to have two groups using body percussion and vocals and two using distinctly different-sounding instruments, such as woodblocks in one and drums in another.

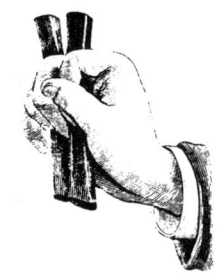

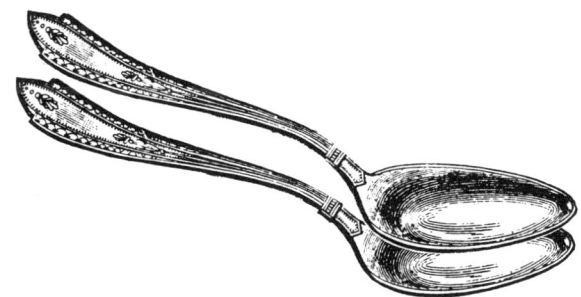

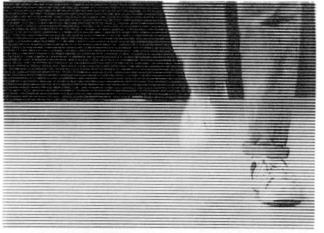

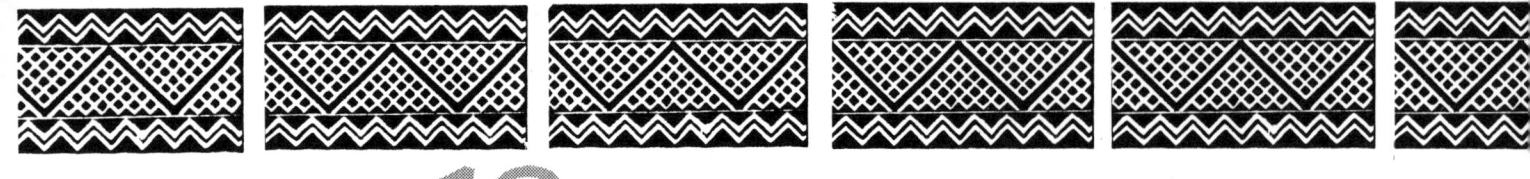

18 COMBINATION 2

Background

In this game, four groups are formed and within each group everyone is involved in simple rhythm constructions (based on a development process) and in the option to improvise rhythms and solos. A synopsis of the form is as follows:

- Four groups are formed, each with a different number cycle.
- Each group has it's own unique "sound character."
- Each group develops a sequence of four rhythms out of the pulse.
- As each group develops its set of rhythms, it incorporates sounds from each of the other groups into the rhythmic patterns.
- Improvising soloists (one at a time from each group) emerge to challenge one another against the accompaniment rhythms of the four groups.
- To end, groups without a soloist withdraw in their own time.

The notated rhythm examples and the suggestions for movement present a challenge that is different from the other exercises in this book. With a bit of practice, this game is easily turned into a performable piece.

Activity Sequence

1. Divide the number of performers (at least 12), into four groups and give (or have each group choose) a number from a consecutive number sequence. (Use the sequence 3, 4, 5, 6 to start, as these numbers are the basis for the notated rhythm examples that follow. Once the system is clear, any other set of consecutive numbers can be tried.)

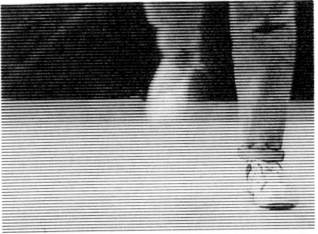

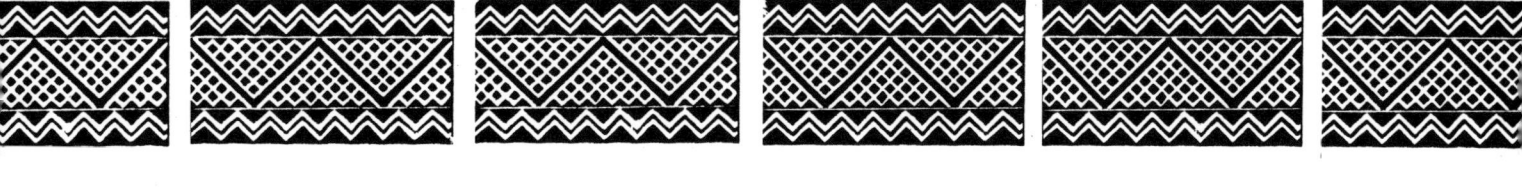

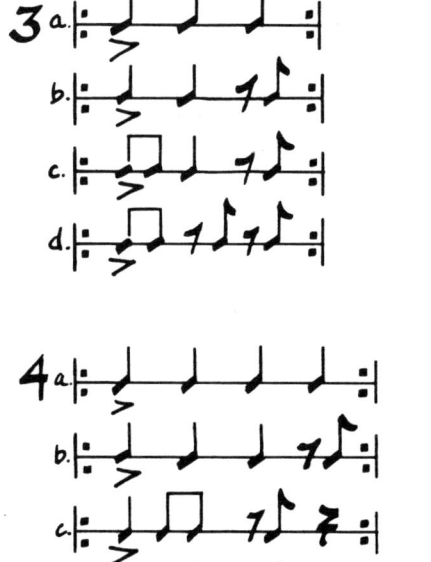

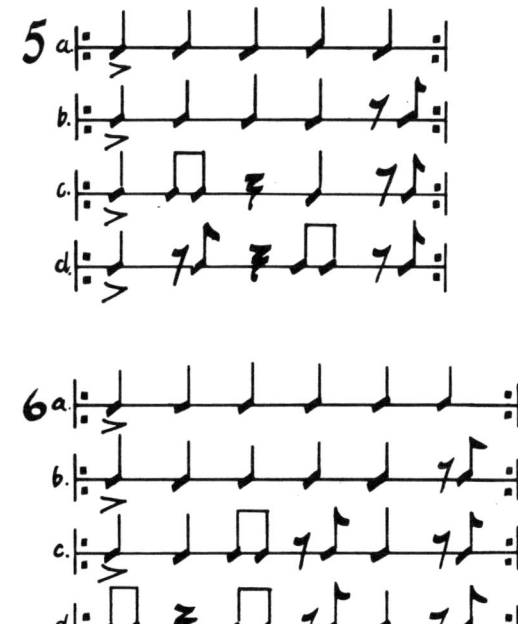

2. Establish the side-to-side foot stamp and run through the notated rhythm sequences with the whole group in the call-and-response style. (Repeat each rhythm of each set four times, and have everybody echo each repeat as in *Call and Response*.)

3. Give (or get each group to choose) a "sound character," i.e., one of the hand or voice sounds listed below.
   whoo/ha (voice)
   chih/chah (voice)
   hoh/hey (voice)
   yah/yoh (voice)
   clap hands
   flick fingers
   slap thighs
   slap chest and/or backside

4. Get each group to go off into a separate corner to rehearse its set of rhythms with its appropriate sound. A leader for each group should be appointed at this stage. (Each group can also devise its own foot-stamping pattern appropriate to its number cycle. *Note:* This is optional.)

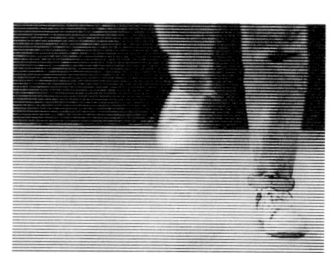

5. Get everyone back (in their groups) into one large circle and explain the game procedure as follows:

   - Each group performs in a semi-circular shape with a leader at one end.

   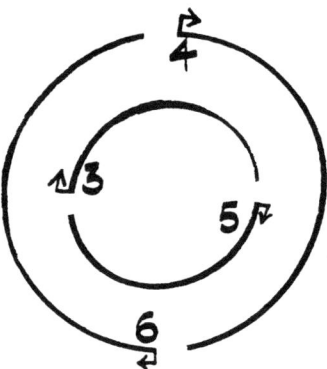

   The leader role may be swapped between players once the rhythm group stage is underway. Anyone wanting to take on this role indicates his intention by moving into an end position.

   - There are three playing roles for each group during the game: pulse group, rhythm group, and soloist.

   - Pulse group stage: Everyone begins with the side-to-side foot-stamping pattern. The leader of each group establishes the group sound in unison with the foot stamp, and optionally, the group foot-stamp pattern appropriate to the number cycle. Others in the group follow suit one by one along the line.

   - Rhythm group stage: Each set of rhythms evolves from the pulse, with each new rhythm in the sequence building on the one previous, and getting progressively more complex. Leaders in their own time begin the first rhythm pattern of their set (accented pulse rhythm), and the rest of the groups follow suit, imitating it one after another. The leaders in their own time move onto the second rhythm, gradually imposing it over the pulse. As each leader switches to a new rhythm, he incorporates into it a new sound (taken from one of the other groups). The rest of the groups follow suit one after another, and so on through to the fourth rhythm. Therefore the rhythms from 1 to 4 in each set progress from a pulsed cycle of one sound in the first rhythm, to an increasing mixture of the sounds made by the four groups in the second, third, and fourth rhythms.

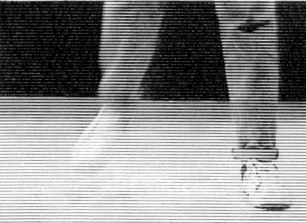

GROUP ONE   : RHYTHM CYCLE 3 :   WHOO/HAH
GROUP TWO   : RHYTHM CYCLE 4 :   CLAP HANDS
GROUP THREE : RHYTHM CYCLE 5 :   YAH/YOH
GROUP FOUR   : RHYTHM CYCLE 6 :   SLAP CHEST

RHYTHM CYCLE 4.

PULSE GROUP STAGE

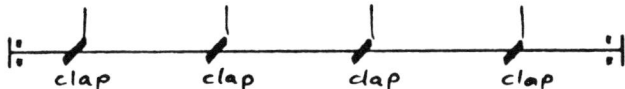

RHYTHM GROUP STAGE

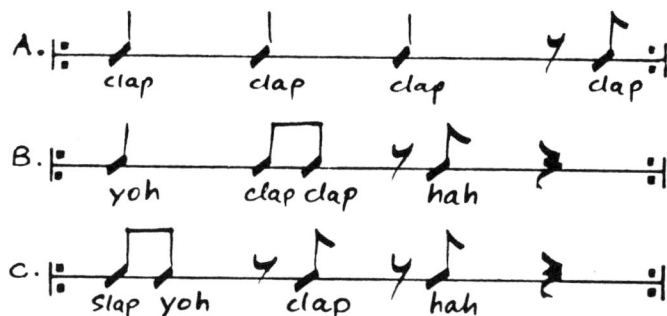

Each group goes through the process of changing its rhythms and accumulating sounds at its own speed, until it arrives at the last rhythm of the set. (This stage takes a bit of practice so be patient.)

- Soloist stage: Soloists are individuals (no more than one at a time) from each group, who are motivated to solo once the final rhythm in the set is reached. Only two soloists can ever be playing at any one time. A soloist can use any combination of sounds, from voice, body, or portable instrument. As soon as a soloist begins, the other players in his group return to the pulse rhythm stage and count and finger-click (or clap) the pulse cycle in a unison accompaniment to the soloist.

- The other groups maintain their rhythm cycles, until one of their group begins a challenge solo. After a brief confrontation, the first soloist gives way and stops.

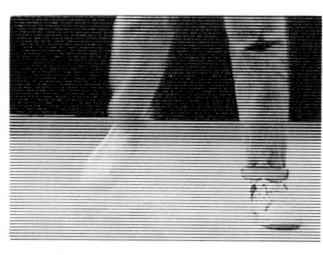

- The group relating to the new soloist now becomes accompanist and quietly counts and finger-flicks its pulse cycle.

- The displaced soloist and group resume the last rhythm of their set—or one improvised on the spot—with the ex-soloist establishing it (as new leader) and the rest of the group imitating until a new soloist emerges. This shifting of roles continues for as long as there are willing soloists.

6. To end, non-soloist groups can agree to stop and withdraw rather than put up new soloists, leaving it to the remaining soloist and pulse groups to run out of steam and exit in their own time. Alternatively, when there are no more soloists forthcoming, each group can retreat or exit in full rhythm and movement.

Developments

- Some movement possibilities: Movement will make this game more interesting visually if it is performed. Try having the two circles constantly on the move, in opposite directions, with the groups turning inward or outward as leaders signal. Don't lose the unison foot stamp. Soloists use the space between the circles to move freely around in while they solo.

- For complete independence of each subgroup, try a four-circle formation of the movements. Each group can then freely choose to move left or right (signaled by a leader) and turn in or out for soloist confrontations or whatever.

- Try doubling the number of soloists playing at any one time.

- Try devising alternative rhythm cycle sets (4, 5, 6, 7; 5, 6, 7, 8; 6, 8, 9, 12) and composing rhythm sequences in the style notated for 3, 4, 5, 6.

Points to note and/or discuss

- Once the game system has been sorted out, leaders in each group might devise their own B, C, and D rhythms spontaneously.

- Suitable signals for whenever there's a change in leader.

- Overall dynamics in relation to solos, and also between one group and another.

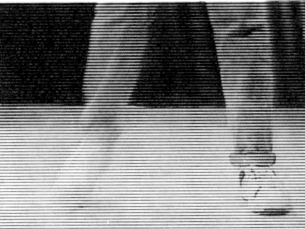

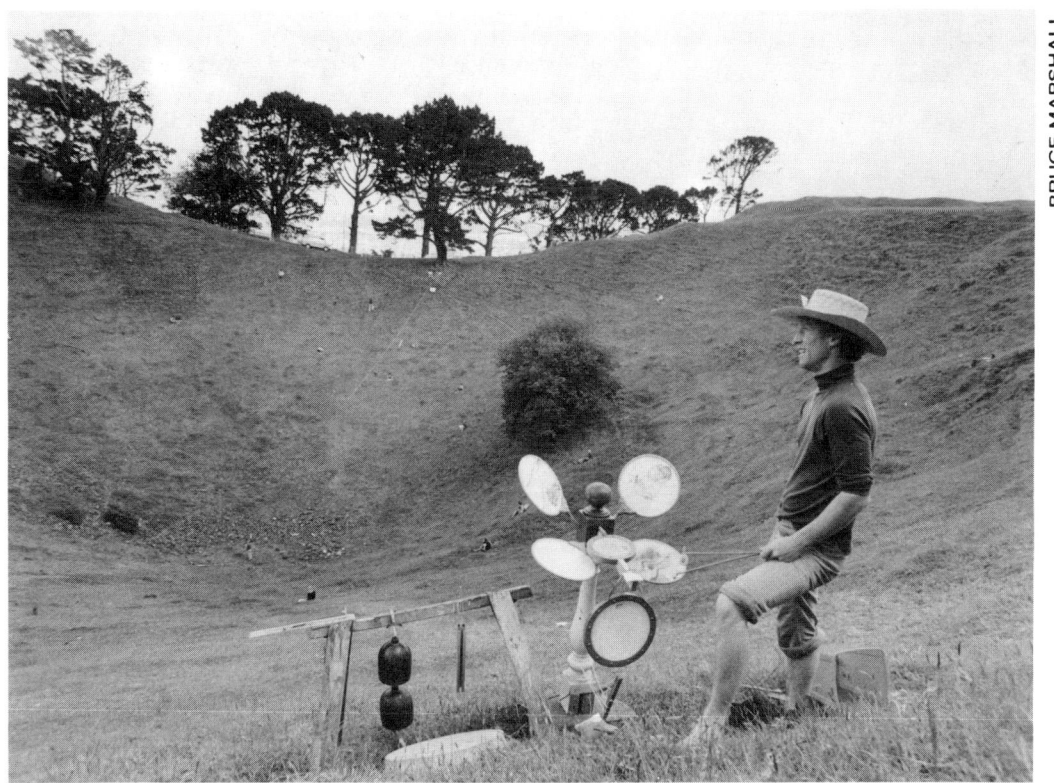

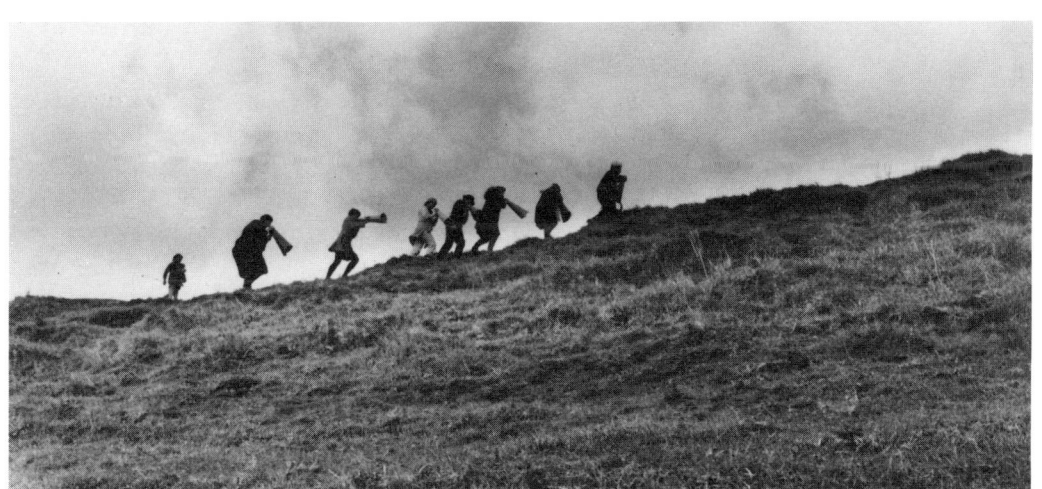

The basic ideas for Combination 2 come from a piece called "Crater Drumming" performed once as part of Solar Plexus, a dawn-to-dusk drumming event held each winter solstice in Maungawhau Crater (Mt. Eden), Auckland City.

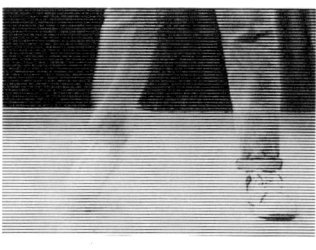

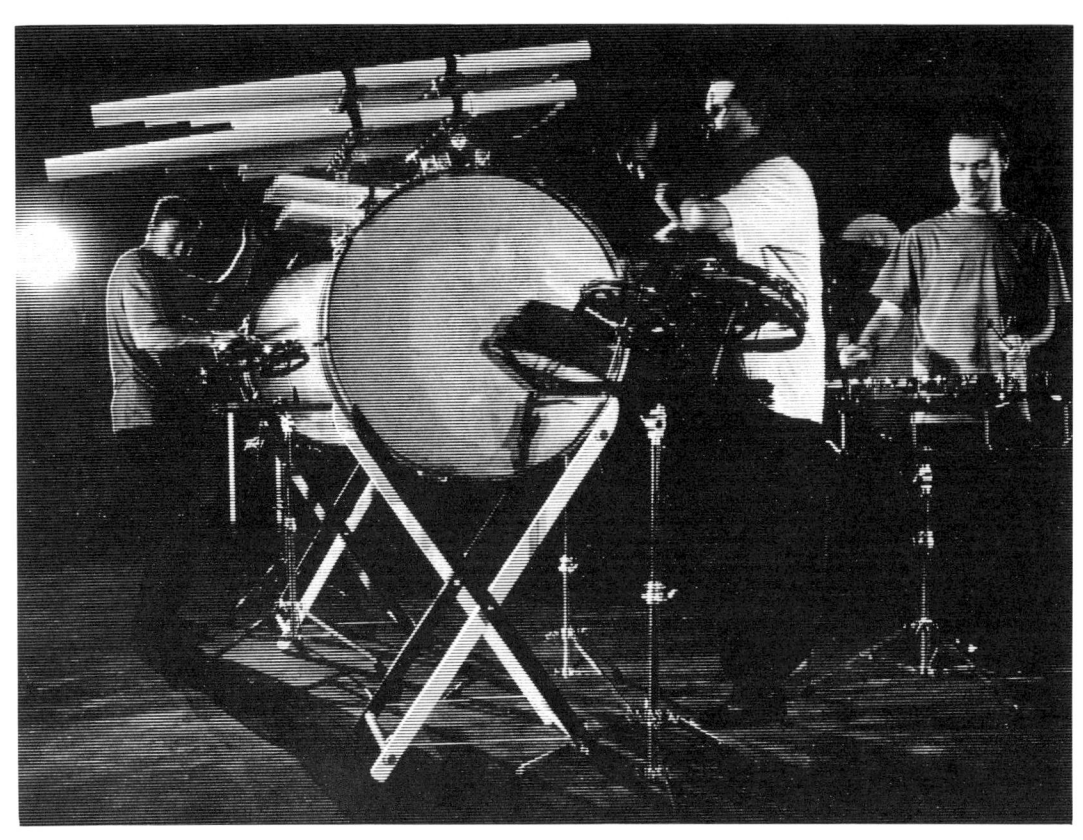

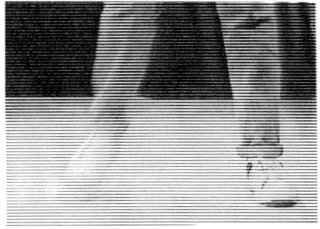

56

APPENDIX 1
A GLOSSARY OF COMMON RHYTHM AND MUSICAL TERMS

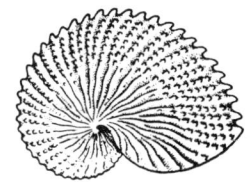

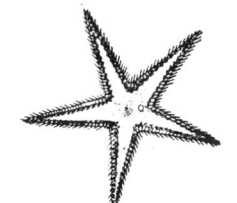

accelerando: gradually getting faster.

ad lib: the liberty to improvise.

beat: (see also *pulse*) a measurement of musical time, the duration of which varies according to the tempo. In notated music, beat can be indicated by the "time signature," e.g., a 4/4 measure has 4 fundamental beats; a 3/8 measure, 3; and a 2/2 measure, 2. The upper figure shows the number of beats in a measure and the bottom figure, the value of the beat or pulse. Music said to have "beat" is music where a rhythmic pulse is distinctive and regular.

canon: (or round) a rhythmic/melodic form, usually a song, so structured that when voices enter at specific intervals, repeating the same phrase or tune, the melody or pattern harmonizes with itself. (See voice exercise, Appendix 2, p. 62.)

cross rhythm: the juxtaposition of different rhythms or accents.

cycle: (in the rhythmic sense) equals one unit of a repeating pattern.

de-accelerando: becoming slower.

Dorian mode: one of eight modes or scales derived from ancient Greece, now commonly called "church modes," which exploit the tones of the basic diatonic scale (the white notes on a modern keyboard instrument). The Dorian mode consists of one octave of white notes beginning on D-natural.

downbeat: the first beat of a measure, commonly marked in an orchestra by the down-beat of the conductor's baton. In this book the downbeat of a rhythmic cycle is usually marked with an accent such as a shout, clap, or foot stamp, and sometimes all three.

foot stamp: a regular rhythmic pattern with the feet synchronized with the beat, such as the side-to-side footstamp. In this book the foot stamp is used as a pulse reference (see page 2).

free rhythm: music or action without a strict "pulse" reference (see *Action Loop Game 1*).

harmony: when two or more voices or melodic parts combine in a way that is musically significant. Harmony is often referred to as the "vertical" in musical structure, while melody pertains to the "horizontal."

hemiola: a Baroque term for note values standing in the relationship of 3 to 2, that is, alternating sections of duple and triple meter, 2 x 3 pulse and 3 x 2 pulse. Example:

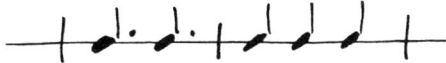

This is a common rhythmic device in much African and Latin music.

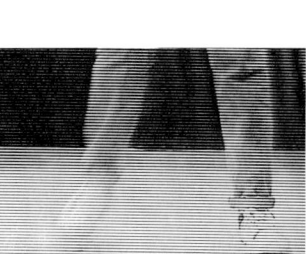

hocket: the on/off sharing of a rhythmic and/or melodic line between two or more players, one part having a rest when the other has a note (see *Hocket* and *Ons and Offs* games).

key: the dominant note(s)—or tonal center—in a piece of music, the most important note being called the "keynote". Key relates to scale, in that for every scale there is a corresponding key and key signature.

loop: a repeating cycle of sounds or movements (see *Action Loop Games*)

meter: the number of beats in a cycle or "measure." The meter of a composition is usually indicated by its "time signature." *Basic meter* types are *Duple* (2/2, 2/4, etc.), *Triple* (3/2, 3/4, 3/8, etc.), *Common* (4/2, 4/4, etc.), and *Compound* (6/8, 12/8, 9/8, etc.). Odd-numbered time signatures higher than 3, such as 5/4, 7/8, etc., are sometimes termed *irregular* meter.

multiple meter: (poly-meter) the simultaneous use of two or more meters, as in most of the exercises in this book.

octave: a scale of twelve consecutive semi-tones (or 8 notes of a normal diatonic scale). Also, an interval from one note to the nearest note (higher or lower) that has the same letter name.

off-beat: a note that falls between two on-beats (see *Ons and Offs.*)

on-beat: a note synchronized with a beat.

ostinato: a short rhythmic/melodic phrase that is repeated persistently, and that can be used to provide accompaniment. (See *Ostinatos and Solos.*)

pentatonic: a scale consisting of 5 tones. There are many forms of pentatonic scales that occur throughout the world, especially in Asia but also in Celtic and other cultures. The most common pentatonic scale uses 5 steps of a diatonic scale: 1, 2, 3, 5, 6. The same scale is represented by the black notes on a piano.

phase: in rhythmic phase/out of rhythmic phase. In-phase: where two or more parts are in synch with each other. Out of phase: where a similar part moves out of synch and into a different relationship (as in *Ons and Offs* and the canon singing exercise, p. 62).

phasing: where one part moves incrementally past another by gradually changing speed and then restabilizing. A term coined by American composer Steve Reich to describe a rhythmic process he devised, based on the slightly different speed rates of analog tape recorders.

poly-rhythm: conflicting rhythms performed simultaneously, often the result of combining different meters (see *Combination 2*).

pitch: the relative high or low frequency of a sound. The key in which a song or piece is set is one of the determining factors of pitch.

process music: where a gradually changing process can be audibly and sometimes visually observed in a performance. A term devised to describe the early minimalistic music of La Monte Young, Terry Riley, Phil Glass, and more particularly, Steve Reich.

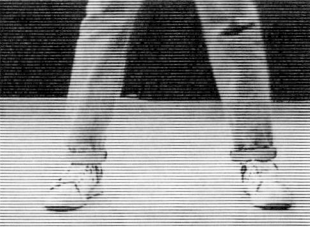

pulse: the steady, regular beat that can be identified in most rhythmic music. The pulse note may be of any time value. It is most commonly a quarter-note, eighth-note, or half-note, and is usually indicated musically by the bottom number of a time signature. The pulse provides a regular anchor for everything else, and in this book the foot stamp serves this purpose.

resultant rhythm: the pattern that results from two interlocking parts played together, e.g., 2 against 3, 3 against 4, etc. (see *Odds and Evens*).

rhythm: from the Greek "to flow," in it's broadest sense a pattern—often regular and repeating—of actions or events (musical or otherwise) that exist in time, e.g., the seasons, phases of the moon, tides, days of the week, diurnal rhythm, circadian rhythm, corporeal rhythm, musical rhythm, etc. There are three aspects to rhythm: time, movement, and regularity or irregularity. In this book, rhythm is mostly characterized by repeating patterns of beat, pitch, and movement, with a regular pulse reference.

syncopation: the accenting of weak beats in relation to strong beats. Where beats and off beats are combined in interesting ways. Syncopation also occurs when different meters are combined together, e.g., 3/4, 4/4, and 5/4. Syncopation can also be a result of "hemiola," where a time signature such as 6/4 can be felt and played in two different ways at once.

tempo: the speed of the beat (pulse) in a piece of music.

time signature: the sign that indicates the meter of a piece of music. Usually 2 numbers, the upper representing the number of beats per bar and the lower one the time value of each beat.

tone: (1) the quality of a musical sound. (2) a pitch interval consisting of two semi-tones, e.g., C-natural to D-natural.

tonic sol-fa: A system used mainly by singers to name the notes in the diatonic scale: doh, ray, me, fa, so, la, ti, doh.

tuned percussion: percussion instruments on which notes of "definite" pitch can be played, e.g., marimba, xylophone, etc.

untuned percussion: percussion instruments on which sounds of "indefinite" pitch can be played, e.g., shakers, rattles, clavés, etc.

up beat: usually the beat preceding the main accent (the downbeat) and often referred to as the weak beat. Not to be confused with off beat.

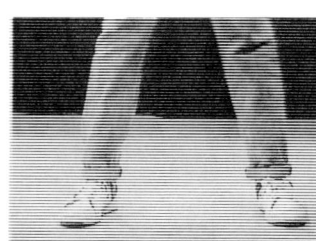

APPENDIX 1A
A GUIDE TO UNDERSTANDING THE MUSICAL NOTATION IN THIS BOOK

Comparative Table of the Relative Value of Notes

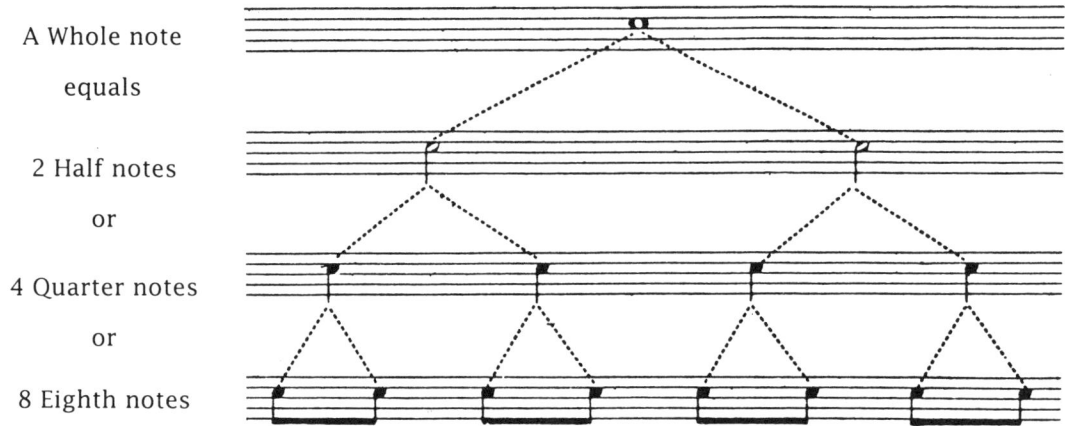

A Whole note equals

2 Half notes or

4 Quarter notes or

8 Eighth notes

Rests

Instead of a note a *rest* of equal value can be placed.

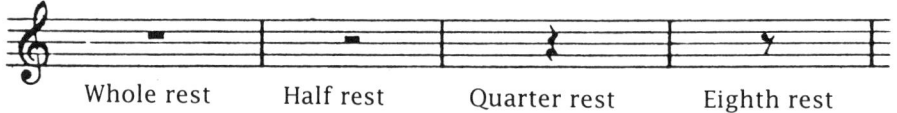

Whole rest   Half rest   Quarter rest   Eighth rest

In rhythmic notation, when pitch is unimportant, one line can be used for each strand of rhythmic information. If nonspecified pitches are used, notes can be placed on the line and above and below (see examples in *Stamping 1*), or two or three lines can be used, as in Appendix 4, *Composing Rhythms*.

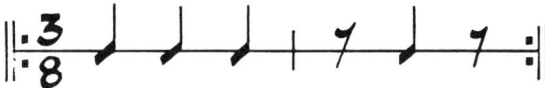

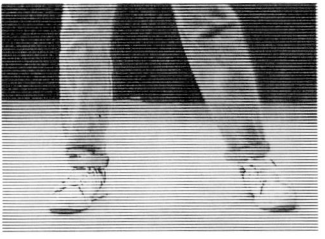

60

In the preceding diagram, the pattern consists of two bars of 3/8, with double barlines at each end to indicate beginning and end of pattern. The two dots at the beginning and end of the pattern indicate that the rhythm is to be repeated over and over. The numbers at the start of the line indicate the time signature, and the notes used are eighth notes.

Where pitch information *is* important, a stave of five lines is used. In this book all notation is written in the treble clef, i.e., in the region above and immediately below middle C on the piano.

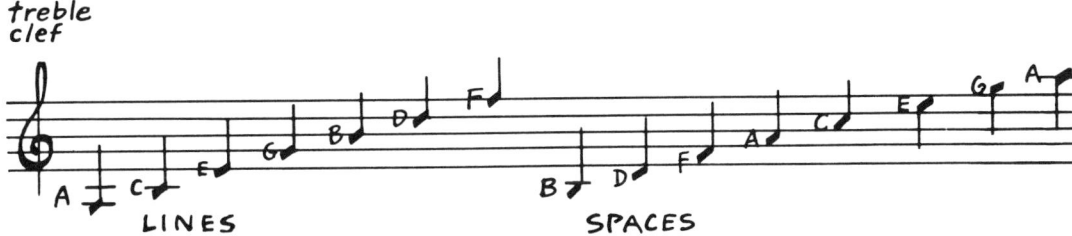

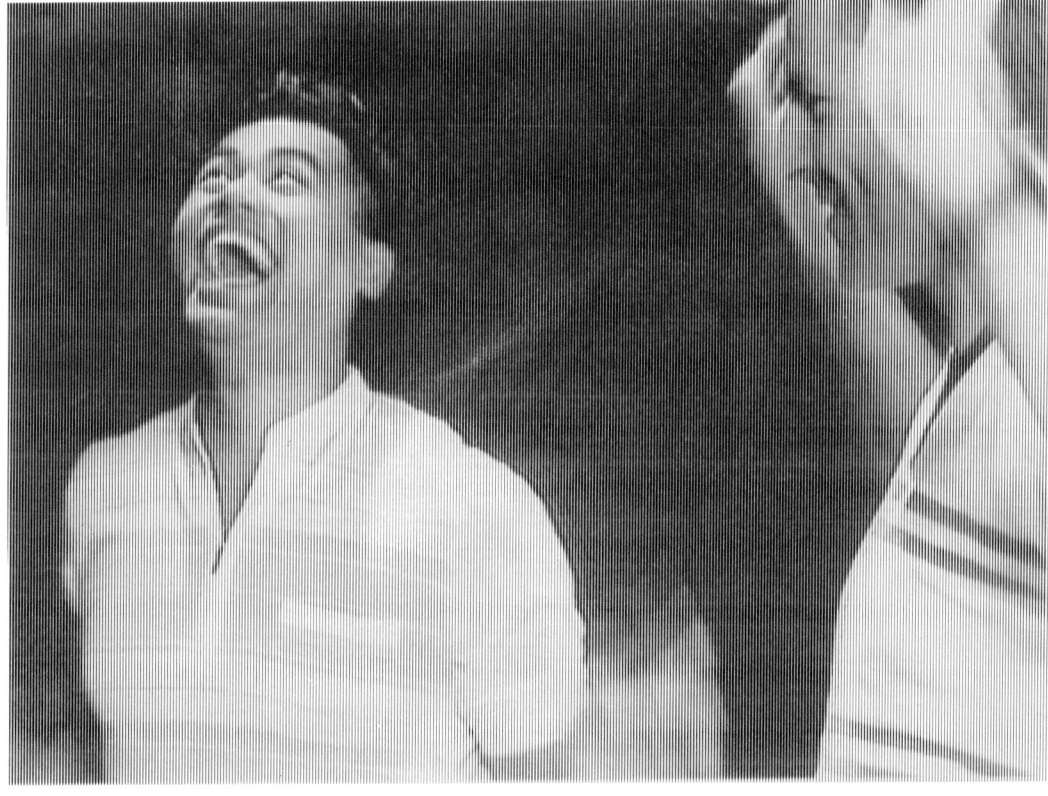

61

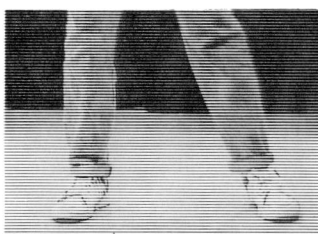

APPENDIX 2
VOCAL WARM-UPS

Vocal Warm-Up 1

Divide the group up into three and give each group one note of a major triad: tonic, third, and fifth. The example given is in the key of F major.

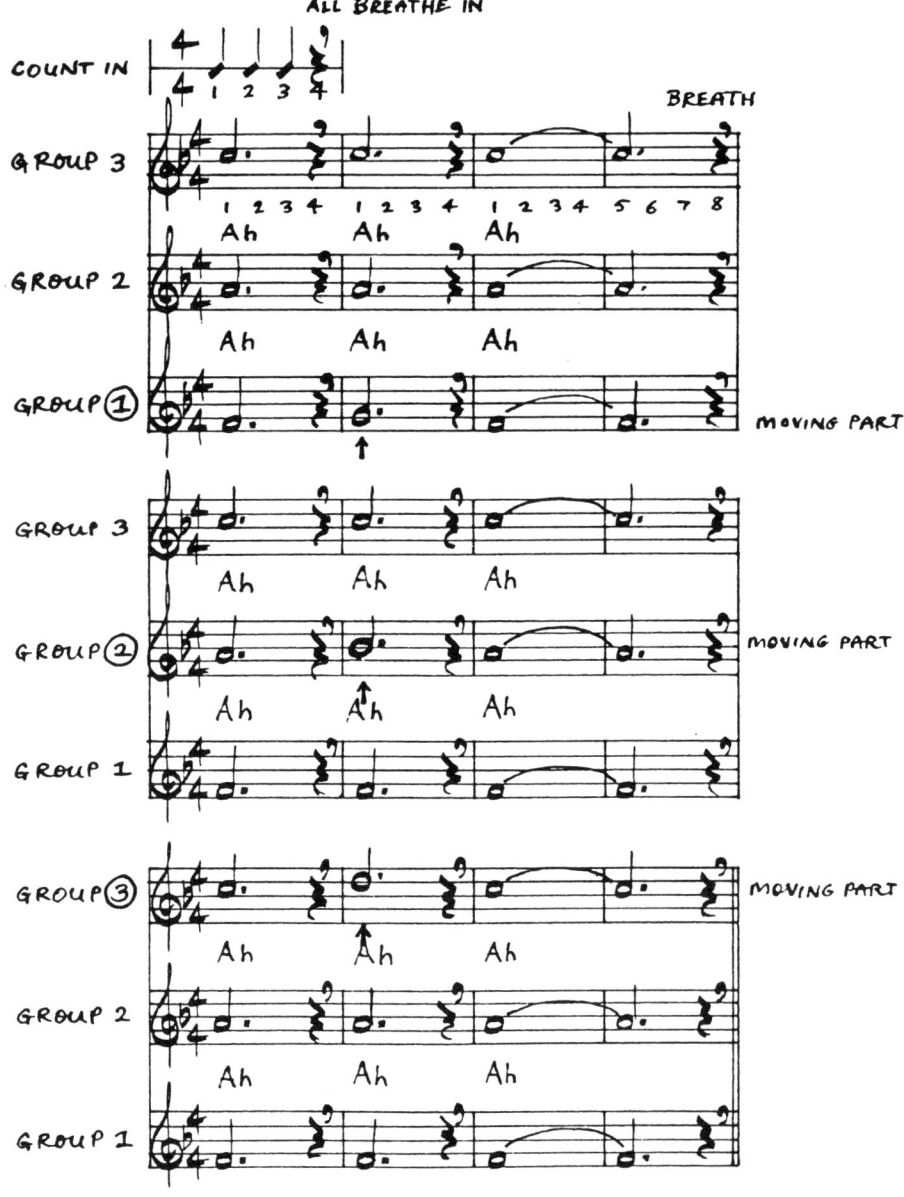

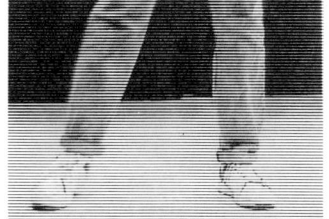

Keep a steady pulse (the side-to-side foot shuffle works well) and encourage the group to listen to the "new" chords (the ones in bar 2) as well as to the long held chords (bars 3 and 4).

Everyone will hear the way the group naturally "tunes" the familiar major chord. By the end of bar 4 the triad will be more in tune than at the start of bar 3.

This is a good exercise to help build the confidence of those who have never sung before. It's possible to have a good group sound quite quickly.

When the three groups have sung through the exercise once (to the end of bar 12), move the triad up one whole tone and repeat the whole process without stopping. When the group gets good at it, move the triad up or down a chosen scale according to the range of voices available.

For variety, try the exercise using minor chords, or as follows:

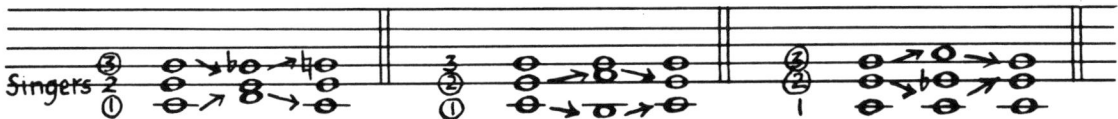

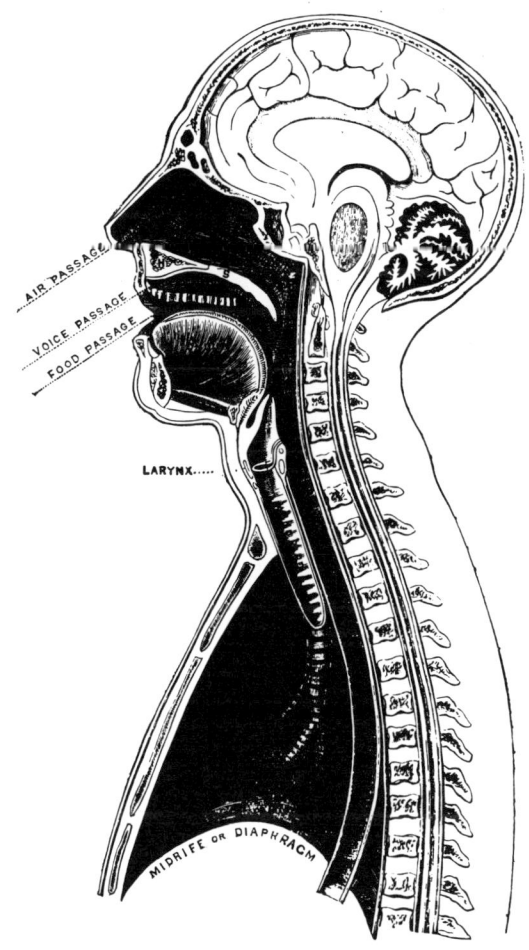

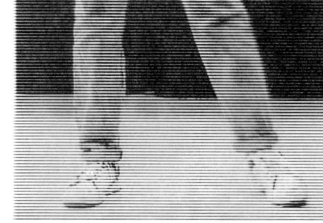

Vocal Warm-Up 2

This vocal exercise, although useful as a warm-up and tune-up, also introduces part singing via simple canon procedure. Thanks, Gloria Jenkins.

Activity sequence

1. Demonstrate the beginning of the following and then have everyone sing the sequence in unison, using either numbers (as illustrated) or tonic solfa.

    1
    1,2,1
    1,2,3,2,1
    1,2,3,4,3,2,1
    1,2,3,4,5,4,3,2,1
    1,2,3,4,5,6,5,4,3,2,1
    1,2,3,4,5,6,7,6,5,4,3,2,1
    1,2,3,4,5,6,7,8,7,6,5,4,3,2,1

    8
    8,7,8
    8,6,7,8
    8,6,5,6,7,8,
    8,7,6,5,4,5,6,7,8
    8,7,6,5,4,3,4,5,6,7,8
    8,7,6,5,4,3,2,3,4,5,6,7,8
    8,7,6,5,4,3,2,1,2,3,4,5,6,7,8
    1

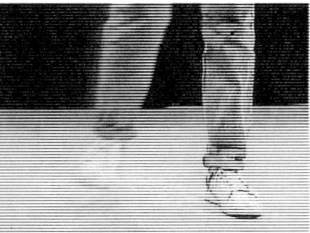

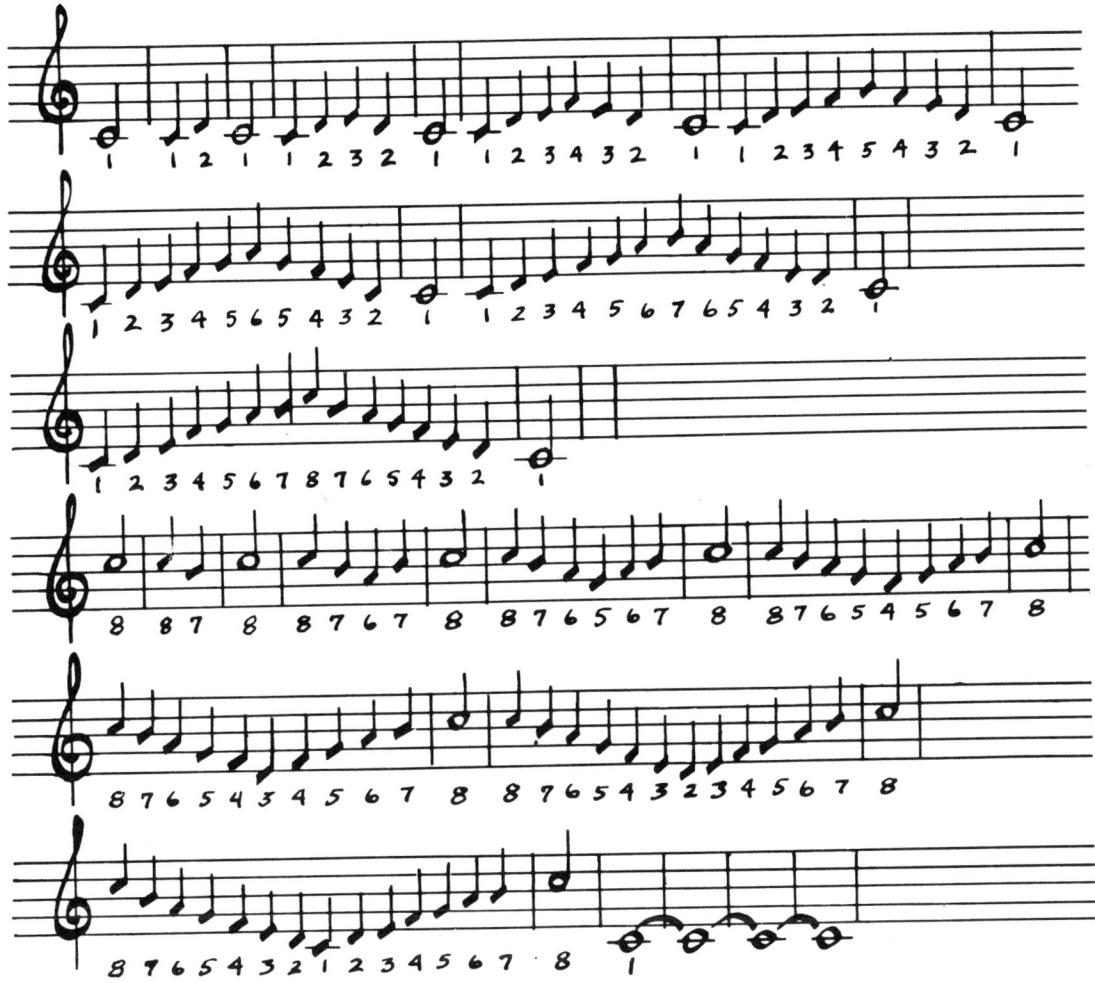

2. Next, divide the group in half, establish a quarter beat pulse and after starting the first group off, start the second group one half beat later, and (in canon) run through the complete sequence.

3. Divide the group in four and do the same thing, starting each group off one half beat after the other.

4. Subdivide further. This canon will work with as many subdivisions as you like, providing everyone stays in tune.

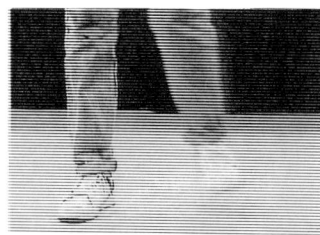

APPENDIX 3
DEVELOPING ON/OFF SINGING

Background

This takes basic singing ideas introduced in *Ons and Offs 1* and *2* several steps further, and develops them into something more like group compositions. Adding vocals takes a little time and presumes you have a basic understanding of scale steps, intervals, and chords, as in the following examples in the key of D minor.

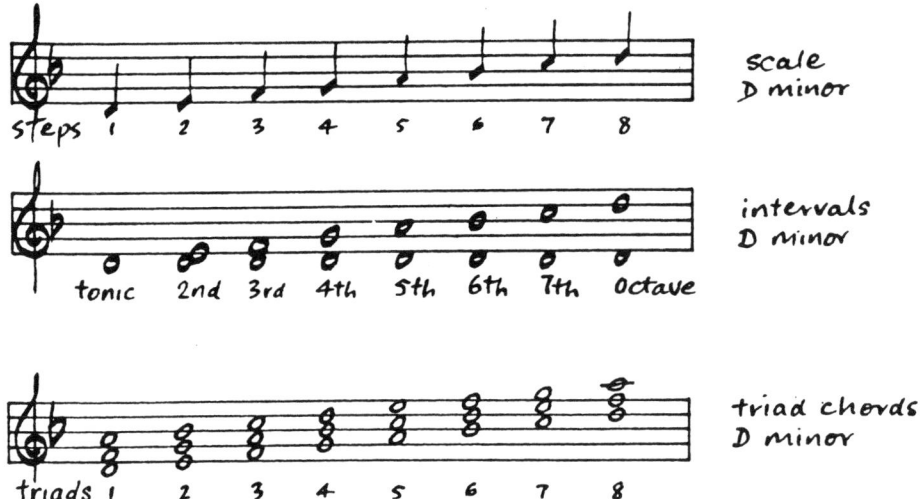

Activity sequence

1. Get the group into a circle and divide in half. Begin the side-to-side foot stamp and the unison on/off clapping in 4/4.

2. Add bar length open fifths as follows (example only):

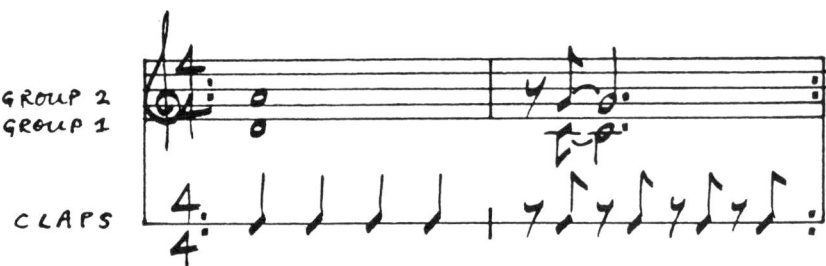

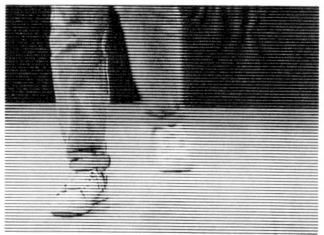

The interval between the open fifths of D minor to C major is one scale step (a whole tone). Demonstrate these intervals by singing or playing the pitch-pairs alternately: A to G, D to C.

3. The next stage develops harmony. Each group learns to move their 2-bar/2-note phrase from a given starting point up or down the scale in whole or semi-tone steps, as dictated by the scale (or mode), in this case D minor.

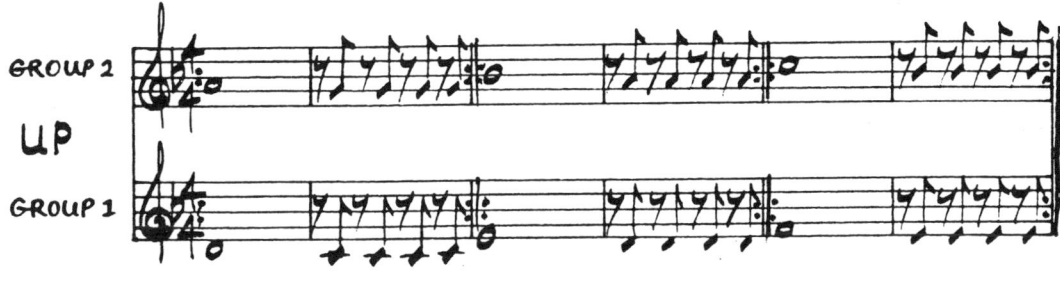

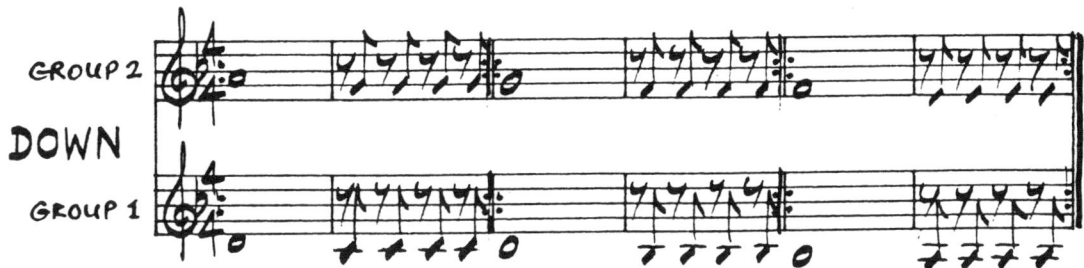

The groups will soon observe that by shifting the pitch-pairs in this way, only one of the two notes changes. Going up the scale one step, the note of the first bar gets transferred to the second bar of the next pitch-pair. Going down, the note of the second bar becomes the note of the first bar in the next pitch-pair.

4. Now go back to the on/off clapping exercise. Two signals are necessary—one to signal "going out" and the other to indicate pitch direction up or down. At this stage one person can easily signal both changes, but the group needs plenty of warning. The best place for signals—"go out," pitch, or both—is at the start of the second bar, the "off" half of the cycle.

   Get the two groups to clap the on/off cycle in unison, but independently move pitch-pairs up and down the scale to produce shifting harmonies. Then go out (one group against the other) independently, shifting rhythms and pitch-pairs, but this time encourage everyone to also practice the four suggested vocal variations (see *Ons and Offs 1*) so they get used to doing several things at once. (Being able to vocally accent onbeats and offbeats in a cycle is important later.)

5. Divide the large group into four subgroups, as in *Ons and Offs 2*, where there are four subgroups (paired) and two time signatures. Each pair of subgroups should be in close proximity to aid hearing the harmonic result from the singing (interlocked

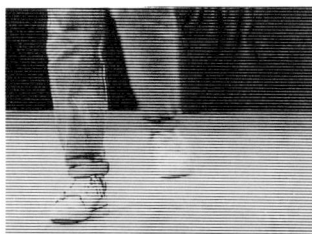

circles are good). Within each "group," one signaler common to both subgroups will indicate pitch changes, (relative to what the other "group" is doing), and each subgroup will have it's own signaler to go out. (Note that it's best to signal a pitch change when both subgroups are in rhythmic unison.)

The combination of rhythm and pitch changes can now start to make some complex and exciting music. This principle can be applied to three, four, or more groups working in the same or different time signatures, or regularly changing number cycles as in *Ons and Offs 3*.

Pitch ad-libbing by some in each group and/or the addition of soloists on instruments is a further option that can be signaled in and out with a bit of prior planning.

Points to note and/or discuss

- Experiment with your own arrangements. You'll find some to be more effective than others.
- When groups are going out against each other, stick to singing short notes on both on-beats and off-beats. It sounds better.

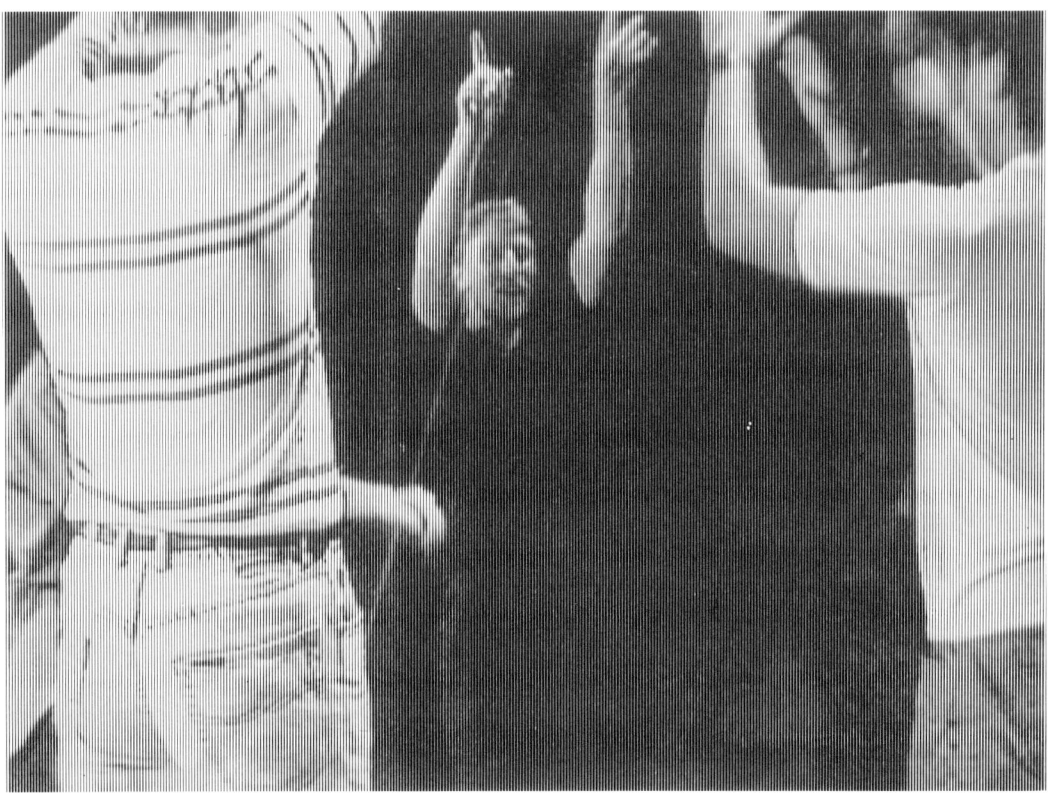

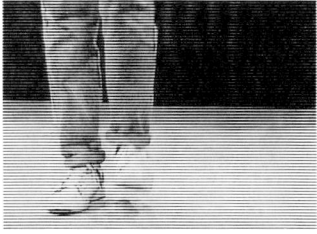

APPENDIX 4
COMPOSING RHYTHMS: A FEW IDEAS

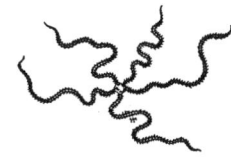
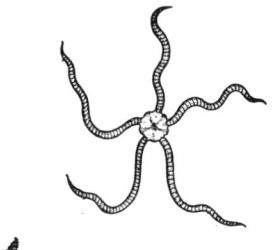
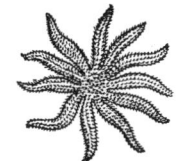
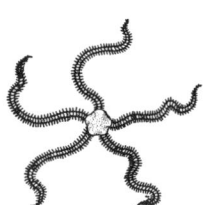

There is a simple law that states: With each consecutive numerical increase of beats in a cycle, the number of possible rhythms that can be made from beat-length notes or rests *doubles*. (In mathematical terms, $2n$. Thanks to Lou Harrison for this simple gem.)

number of beats in a cycle	1	2	3	4	5	6	7	8
number of rhythms available	2	4	8	16	32	64	128	256

For one pulse or beat, there are two possibilities—sounded or silent. For two pulses, four possibilities. For three pulses, eight; for four, sixteen; and so on.

This provides simple rhythm permutations of on-beats and rests with no unit subdivisions, but adding accents and playing the rhythms over different pulse rates expands the possibilities further, for example a 3/8 cell played over an eighth-note, quarter-note, dotted quarter-note, or half-note pulse.

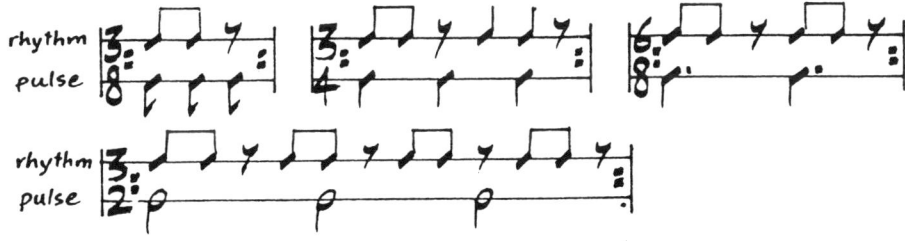

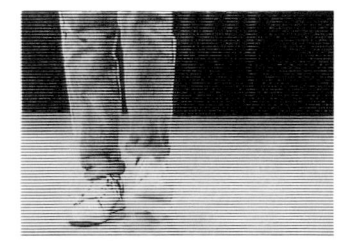

One useful technique for composing rhythms applies the principle of balance:
- alternate left- and right-hand strokes
- pitch distribution across general pitch areas—low, medium, and high.
- pattern inversions, mirror shapes, etc

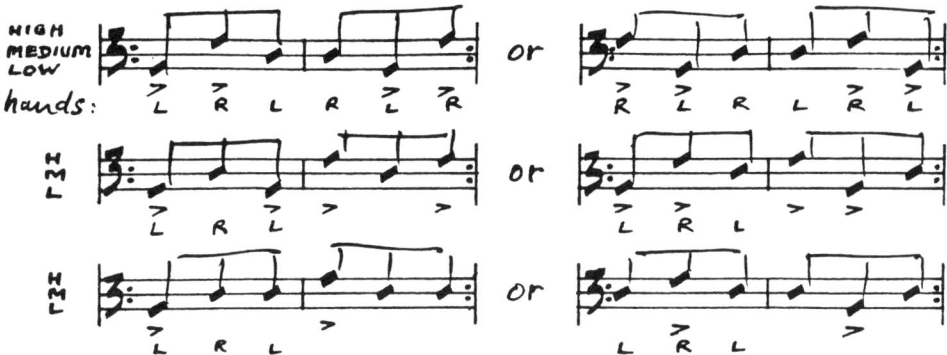

A pattern in 5/8 and one in 8/8

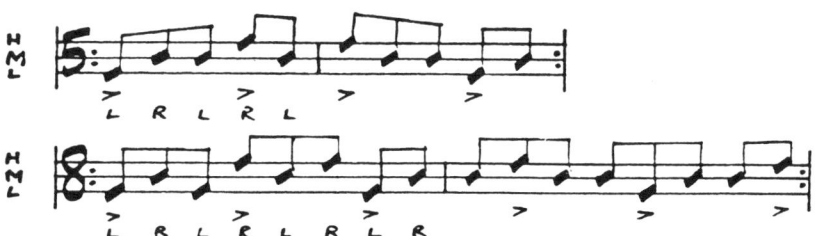

Inversions of these starting on the right hand would sound different again.
Try a progression where you gradually replace notes played with rests of the same value.

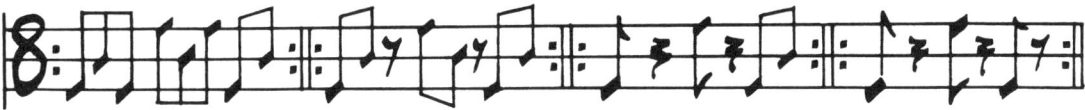

- Rhythms can be sourced and developed from many of the games and exercises in this book, for both composing and playing purposes.
- Try keeping a rhythm notebook for collecting and notating rhythms you see and hear around you. For more ideas along these lines, refer to the VOM notes in Appendix 5
- If you've not yet discovered the world of ethnic music, start listening now. Rhythmic invention in the traditional musics of this planet are an endless and awesome source of inspiration.

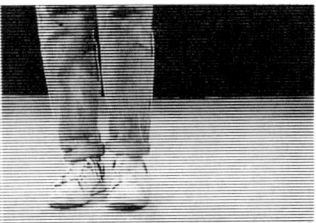

APPENDIX 5
VOM (VARIABLE OCCASION MUSIC) 1972

VOM represents the original impulse and repertoire of From Scratch in 1974 and is included for the purpose of illustrating the background of the rhythm games and exercises in this book.

Background

The VOM manifesto and proposal (1972) was the original probe-and-hatch plan devised for the Auckland Scratch group as an alternative to the loosely structured and largely improvised activities of the then Scratch Orchestra, a New Zealand offshoot of the original London-based Scratch Orchestra founded by English composer Cornelius Cardew.

"Scratch" then was defined as an "instant assembly of enthusiasts" and "orchestra" as "concerted intent"—a definition loose enough to guarantee an open-house attitude for anyone attracted to the ideas. The rhythm stress implicit to the VOM proposal prompted a drift from large-scale group pieces to smaller scale tightly structured rhythm works and to the formation in 1974 of the first From Scratch group, a nucleus of four untrained musician/performers from backgrounds as varied as the visual arts, journalism, and anthropology.

VOM is essentially accompaniment music of rhythmic pattern and texture, from which solos (planned and spontaneous) can emerge. The music is a bit like four people walking barefoot, whose individual body movements vary slightly one from another. External influences modulate their motions—gravel, traffic, friends, rain, grass, darkness, etc.—and any talk between them relegates movement to the level of accompaniment. Talk as a mode of solo rides any dimension but is invariably referenced back to things seen and heard while walking.

A feature of our early music was the junk instruments, found and homemade. Players surrounded themselves with an array of clutter, each article selected for its characteristic sound and look. Sound sources matched categories—resonantly short to long, harmonically simple to complex, aurally deep to high—and were mounted or suspended to surround players at floor level.

From the start, visual interest was equal to the music and today this is still the case. Instruments are characterized by their sculptural look and have evolved from being randomly tuned to finely pitched, and from junk to being designed and built.

VOM: A proposition to the scratch orchestra testing ground for consideration under "valuable ideas."

Aim is to incept a flexible and inclusive format for collective music-making—adaptable to any occasion by arranging variables to a given situation—and to extend the concept of scratch music as proposed in the draft constitution for a scratch orchestra.

VOM is both event and non-event music, aimed at being a reflection of cycles observed in the external world. The ideas essentially propose a flexible framework for rhythm, procedure, and instrumentation, the variables for which are suggested by influences from

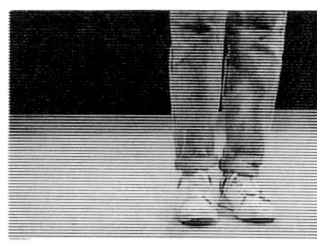

the context or occasion in which the music is to be played, or, variations are composed that determine the variables and establish the occasion—e.g., interim music for a political rally might suggest a title "Muted Thud and Voice Music" plus the appropriate sound sources and procedure, whereas a prearranged format for, say, "Pitched Stone Music," may establish and be the occasion.

All players have a similar rhythm responsibility which might be extended and expanded according to one's lights. Rhythms are derived from an independent or common source. The general procedure is that players begin together or raggedly—slow—to a common pulse or each to his own, gradually increasing pace to a common equilibrium. Players solo as motivated singly or in unison, using the mainstream of rhythm as accompaniment (voices and instruments that emulate the voice are recommended for solos). Players sit, stand, whatever, as instruments and whim permit, in a circular fashion facing inward, extending outward.

Rhythm

Each member of the orchestra should undertake to collect rhythms, notating examples and ideas into a VOM rhythm manual. This should be your personal research book, and as such, can be entered into as you like.

A rhythm is essentially a cycle of beats comprising so many played and so many silent ones. Rhythms can comprise as few or as many units as desired, and the collection should constitute a continually expanding variety of shorts and longs—any long rhythm can be dissected into shorts and likewise shorts combined into longs. The manual should serve a practical need in music-making and provide source materials for the composition of variations. Cultivate curiosity and keep the collection in flux.

The following are suggested starting points:

Selected—notated rhythms of personal choice from any source.

Applied—from patterns observed in natural and manufactured phenomena.

Random—from sources where personal choice is minimized, i.e., a selected source but random result, e.g., (1) number systems; (2) event system, where rhythm is the random but cyclic side effect of a repetitive physical event.

External—devices, mechanical, electronic, etc., which produce random or predetermined rhythm.

Plus the inspired and intuitive rhythm improvised spontaneously in accordance with the heart's response. Use discrimination in what you play in a given context.

Implicit to rhythm is action and non-action. Explore this and associated references and keep a tag on findings.

Solos

Anyone moved to make one is qualified. Soloists might do so singly, in unison, apart or in rapport, and spontaneously as they occur. A soloist should make it clear he is in solo by some means—a gesture or other. A solo might be verbal, melodic, gestural, percussive, or a mixture—each occasion may influence the mode of solo and reversely, solos the occasion.

Suggestion: Inspiring and renovating texts selected for the context might provide solo material for performers.

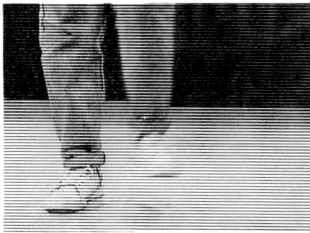

Investigate VOM as a mode of play. Variations influence, to a greater or lesser degree, an overall and personal procedure to which players cultivate versatility. Some simply outline, others fill in detail. Outlines might be applied to more detailed variations, and the more detailed procedures might suggest freer outlines. Submit variations to the orchestra for trial as they come to light.

The following is an exercise and simple example of a rhythmic hub:

Sit in a circle and count off around it, beginning or ending no lower than digit 5, e.g. if there are 8 players numbered 15 to 8, each player's number corresponds to a cycle of rhythm of the same number of beats, for the present silent.

Players begin by sounding 1, 2, 3, or 4 beats only within their cycle—the higher the player's number, the more accents in the cycle; the lower, the less.

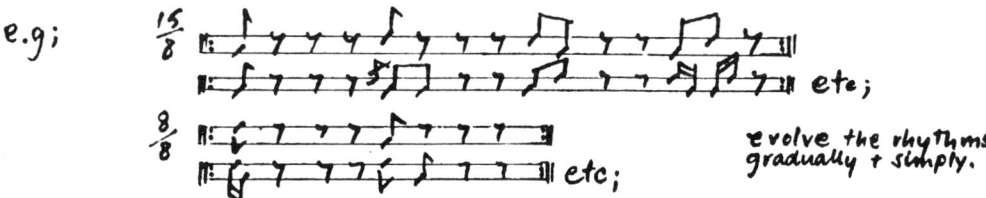

To begin with, play beats by speaking or singing the corresponding number. Intonate all or part of the word freely and keep the word treatment as regular as the rhythm for a given cycle. Independently repeat a cycle of rhythm until it is at ease in the context, and change when you feel it appropriate. Initially you might simply adjust emphasis, exploring various permutations of played beats, and then gradually introduce 1 or 2 new sounds with each subsequent change until you are playing every beat within the cycle. Freely play on or off the beat, and as you change or increase the number of played beats, so you might change or add sound sources. (*Note: This idea was developed into the more "game-like" structures such as Birthday Games 1 and 2.*)

Determine procedure from the following variables:

Ignition
1. The player with highest number begins and the other players commence as their number comes up in the course of another player's rhythm.
2. All begin together at a signal.

Meter
1. a. Adhere to a common pulse.
   b. Keep your own pulse independent of others.
2. a. Begin very, very slowly and slowly increase to a comfortable and collective momentum.
   b. Keep momentum at a constant.

Ending
1. Continue until all appear to be playing completed cycles—await a density peak of sorts and drop out irregularly and independently.
2. Following a density peak, the person who thinks she's last to arrive gives a prearranged signal for an abrupt stop.

Try the same piece substituting vocal sounds and body percussion for the numbers counted—sounds that are an extension of yourself.

Substitute the number system for another. For example:

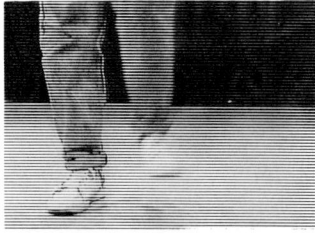

1. Each player draws a square comprising from between 5 to 10 vertical and horizontal columns, i.e., 25, 36, 49, 64, 81, or 100 units to a square. Having decided on size, derive numbers from a random source, e.g., a pack of cards, and fill in the columns. The largest number in a column indicates the length of a cycle. All digits in a given column are played or silent as you decide. Numbers used need not only be between 0 and 9 but also could be between, say, 7 and 20, depending on the cyclic range you want. Play through the columns in any order, playing beats for *all* or a *fraction* of their value; in other words, compose your rhythms using this random system as a starter.

2. Write numbers between 1 and 10 on separate sheets of paper. In successive shuffles take 2, 3, 4, 5, and 6 from the pack until you have a dozen or so variants. The largest number from each draw determines the number of beats in a cycle, and is either silent or accented—the remaining number(s) are played beats; the counts between, silent.

VOM Variations: 1–8

1. All players, prior to beginning, have on hand a selection of different rhythms. Players surround themselves with a wide array of percussion sound sources and begin together to a common pulse, playing very slowly at first and keeping a cycle of sound sources constant to a particular rhythm (change sources as you change rhythm). Gradually and collectively increase the pace, decorating played beats where possible. Drop out individually when a rhythm breaks down with pace.

2. One begins, then others begin in their own time after the player to their left has started—each to his own pulse—striving not to align with others and keeping constant. When firm, align yourself to another player and gradually phase with him. Play like this for as long as you like. Before changing to another rhythm, briefly rest, then continue against any apparent pulse, trying not to align until your cycle is firm—and so you proceed at a fluctuating pace in alternating phases of disorder and alignment. At some time, stop suddenly and solo in an interjectory way. Instrumentation-free. End collectively following a general alignment.

3. On introducing a rhythm, begin by accenting one beat in the cycle only. With subsequent repetitions gradually introduce the remainder until the whole rhythm is stated. Establish it briefly and move on to another rhythm in the same manner. Tempo-free. When you have tired of rhythm, solo exhaustively and drop out.

4. Throughout play, collectively stop and restart as general feeling motivates it. Stop as soon as possible after you notice another player has stopped. Begin in the same way—as soon after another player as possible. Anyone can stop, anyone can start. Impetus for stops and starts must be spontaneous and motivated in response to group feeling. The first one to stop might make it apparent, like freezing, for example. The variation starts and ends similarly; i.e., start as soon after another player as possible and end when no one reignites. Make use of a wide range of percussion sounds favoring rattlings, scratchings, scrapings, clackings, and gentle clash clatter.

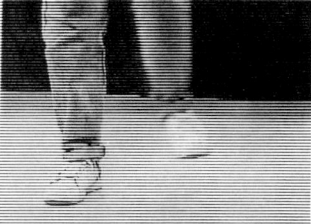

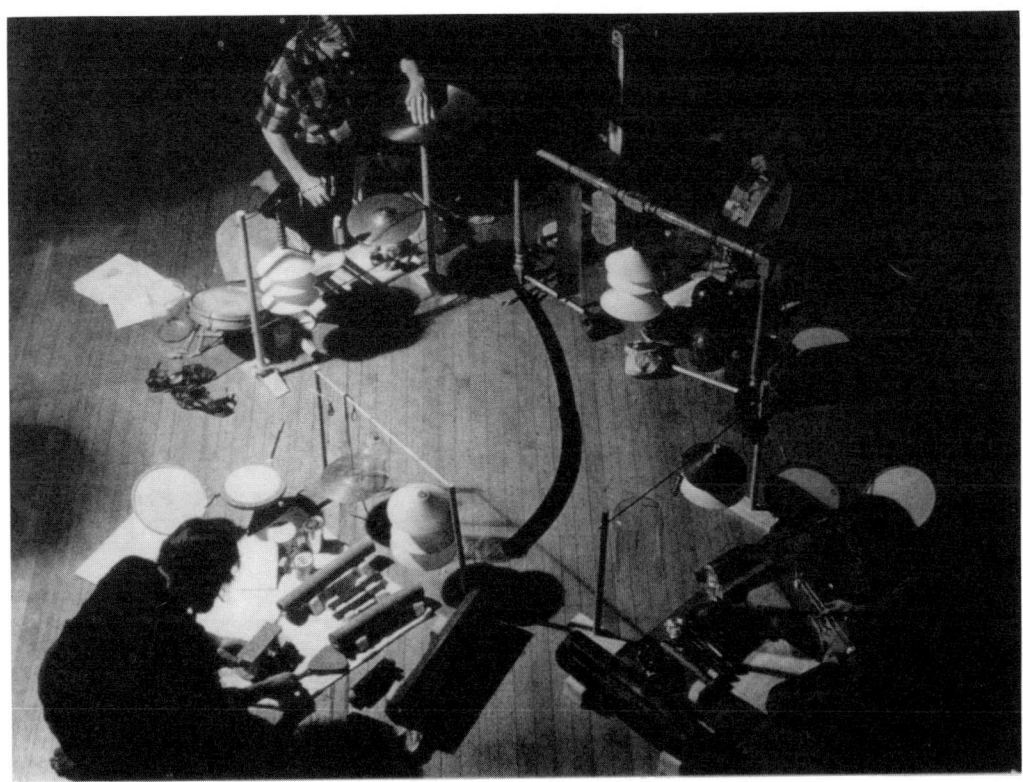

The VOM pieces [particularly 5–8] were the repertoire of *From Scratch*, 1974–75, and were first performed in public at Sonic One (Wellington 1974) and later on in a national campus tour.

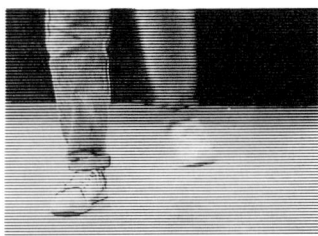

VOM 5 'LOOP MUSIC'

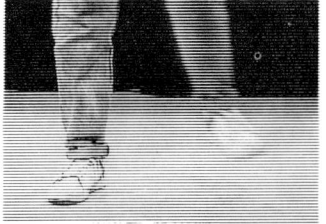

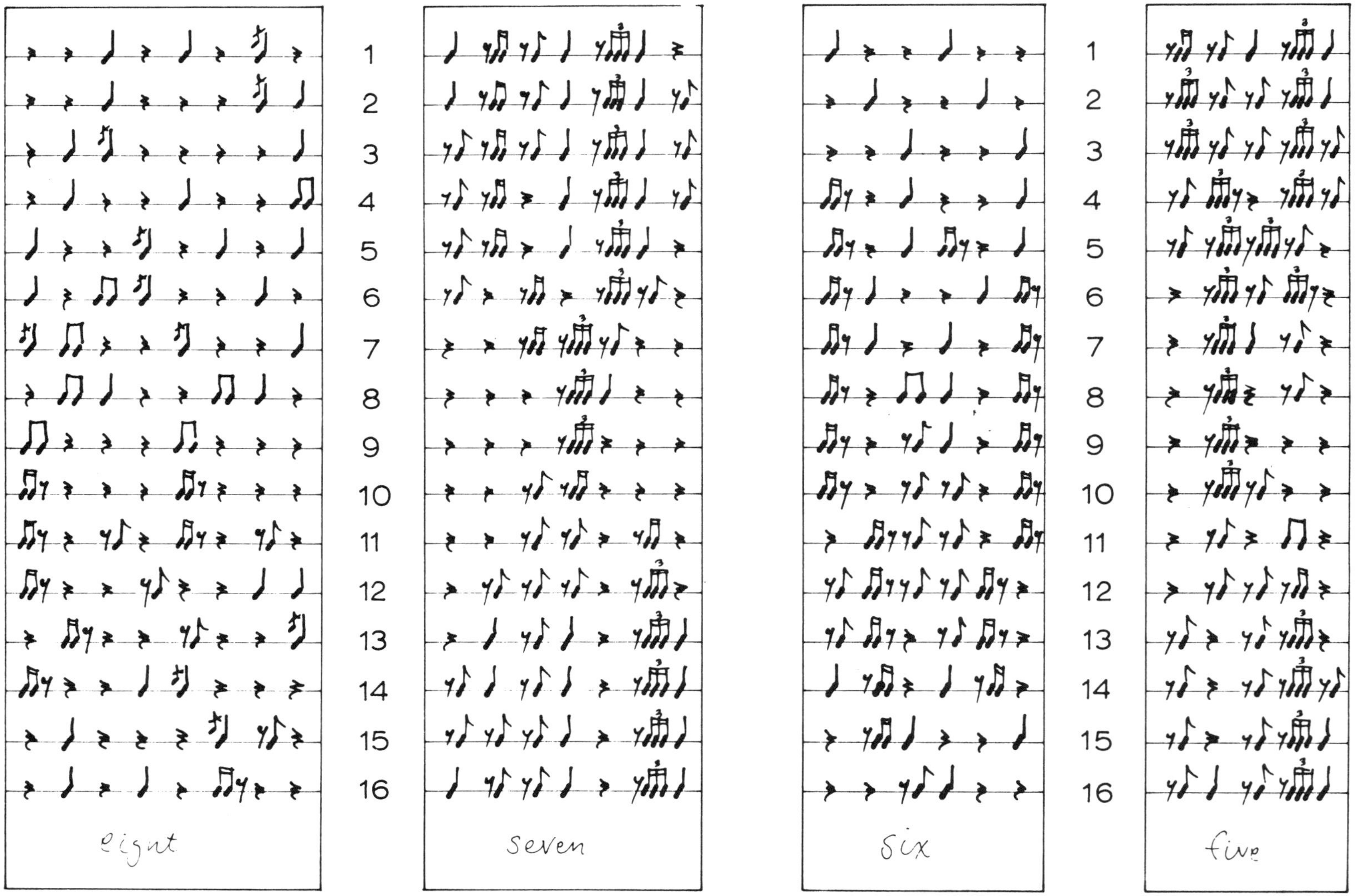

5. **VOM 5: Loop Music**

Notation: There are four sets of rhythmic loops of 5, 6, 7, and 8 beats, respectively. If there are four players, each begins on a different set. If there are more than four, duplicate accordingly.

The piece is cyclic in three ways. First, the rhythm, which you repeat for as long as feels right in the context; second, the set—begin anywhere and end where you began, keeping the direction of progress constant for a given set; and, third, the sets (i.e., all four sets must be played through one of the two directions of progress). Each player works independently through the sets, ending when the 64 loops have been played.

Instrumentation: Each player assembles a wide array of percussion and sound sources (at least 8):

- sonorous to dull
- brittle to solid
- deep to high

For a given set, assign to each basic beat in the cycles 1 or a number of sound sources: e.g., if you are 7 to start, arrange around you 7 sound sources or 7 groups of sound sources that number 1 to 7 from left to right, the way you read the rhythm. Notated notes are played on corresponding sound sources. This basic grouping of sources remains fixed for the time it takes to complete the 16 variants in a set.

As players become skilled, the sound source for each played beat can be selected from anywhere in the array in accord with the collective sound. These then remain fixed for as long as one rhythm is played over and over.

Procedure: Players stand or sit, surrounded by their instruments, in a circle that includes the audience.

Option: One or more circular spaces filled with a variety of instruments are arranged. Any player on completion of a set can move to this space, rearranging the instruments freely for her next set, and leaving her former circle of clutter for another player to move to. If the option is taken, there is no obligation to move on again.

Ignition: Players sit prepared and motionless. No one is elected to begin—one must. All players gear themselves to synchronize entries with the first sound they hear. Or each player sights a sound source of another player's to which he aligns himself and attempts a synchronized entry with the sound from it. No one is elected to begin.

Each player, coincident with her first sound, shouts the number of the set she begins with, and subsequently changes to. Whoever plays 8 is responsible for a pulse, others align to it.

The piece begins very slow, and gradually increases to a comfortable and collective momentum—generally, move without falter through the rhythms, pausing only where essential and indicated. Following a pause, synchronize reentry with another player.

Any player can solo if motivated—voice sounds are recommended. After soloing, pause then continue rhythm where you left off, or begin a new set. (Words, sounds, and gestures appropriate to the occasion should be considered.)

Philip Dadson, Summer '72

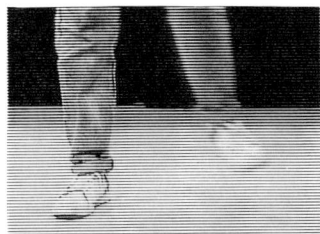

VOM 6. for 3 or 4 percussionists.

A POSSIBLE TRANSITION:

Rhythm	Pattern	Instruments
↓ 3.	♩ ♩ ♪	THREE WOOD
4.	♩ 𝄽 ♩ ♪	TWO WOOD, ONE TIN
5.	♩ 𝄽 ♩ 𝄽 ♪	ONE WOOD, ONE TIN, ONE DRUM
6.	♩ 𝄽 𝄽 ♩ 𝄽 ♪	ONE TIN, ONE DRUM, ONE GONG
7.	♩ 𝄽 𝄽 𝄽 ♩ 𝄽 ♪	TWO DRUMS, ONE GONG
↕ 8.	♩ 𝄽 ♩ 𝄽 ♩ 𝄽 ♩ 𝄽	TWO GONGS, TWO DRUMS,
7.	♪♩ 𝄽 𝄽 𝄽 ♩ 𝄽	TWO GONGS, ONE DRUM
6.	♪♩ 𝄽 𝄽 ♩ 𝄽	ONE GONG, ONE DRUM, ONE TIN
5.	♪♩ 𝄽 ♩ 𝄽	ONE DRUM, ONE TIN, ONE WOOD
4.	♪♩ 𝄽 ♩	TWO TIN, ONE WOOD
↑ 3.	♪♩ ♩	THREE TIN

6. VOM 6: For Three or Four Percussionists

(Note: This piece was one of the more successful. It has a simple structure and is satisfying to play.)

Each player has an assortment of instruments: six medium- to high-pitched, of short resonance from two sources (e.g., wood and tin), and four medium- to low-pitched, of long resonance from two sources (e.g., drums and gongs).

At Rhythm 3, play only instruments of short resonance from one source (e.g., wood), and at Rhythm 8 play only those of long resonance from two sources. In the transition between high and low numbers, make a transition also between sound sources (see the illustration).

To start, the players align themselves as follows: 1 to top 3, 1 to bottom 3, and 1 or 2 to center 8.

Three Players: From the starting point, players move through the rhythms in the direction indicated (8 has an option), ending on the initial rhythm started—8 begins and sets the pulse and the 3s begin soon after in their own time. Speed is moderate to start with, but it may gradually and collectively increase. Dynamics are moderately soft. Change from one rhythm to the next is triggered by 8, who, at his discretion, strikes a signal source (e.g., a cymbal) for the first beat only of each new rhythm. On the signal, players change at completion of the cycle they are on. *(Note: When two players reach 8, one plays on the off beat, except in the case of four players, where two begin in unison at 8.)*

Four Players: Similar procedure to that for three players, except for the two players starting from 8. They move in opposite directions, and one of the two gives signals. The two make a synchronized start, and the 3s follow on the pulse.

When all have moved full circle, the signal player, at his discretion, draws things to a close by playing a short flourish on all or any of his instruments. The others follow suit and end raggedly.

Philip Dadson, '73

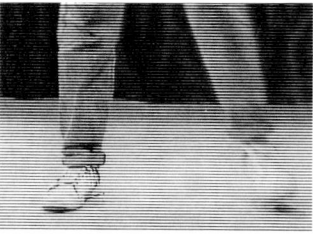

7. **VOM 7: Waxing and Waning Influences: Four Drummers**
(Note: This piece is quite game-like. It needs spontaneity to work. The structure can be adapted to language and gesture, which we often did in the middle of the drumming.)

Sound: There are four sound sources, each source having two pitches:

- wood
- drum
- metal
- gong

Rhythm: There are four rhythm "phases," each with two transition possibilities—from Grey to White or Grey to Black. Grey rhythms are median rhythms. They are the matrices that establish the basic time values for Black and White. Black rhythms are devolved by abstracting sounded beats from the Grey. White rhythms are evolved by unpacking (from sounded and silent beats of the Grey), their more complex rhythmic potential.

Start: Each of the four drummers chooses a separate phase and begins on the grey rhythm within that phase. While playing cycles of this rhythm, the drummer may experiment with all of the four sound sources, with the aim of choosing one. After this choice, the drummer proceeds to develop either the black or the white rhythm within her phase.

Trough: At this point there is not necessarily any waxing influence, though there might be. For example, if three drummers have independently chosen to develop white rhythms, this strengthens the possibility of one white rhythm becoming the dominant influence. The *black* rhythms move toward silence and can actually achieve silence at an individual level, though not at a group level, with one exception (see "Ending" subhead). For each cycle of the grey, one beat is abstracted from the end or the beginning of the grey rhythm.

The *white* rhythms move toward dense sound as beats and groups of beats are detonated from the grey time-value equivalents. As with the black, the process of

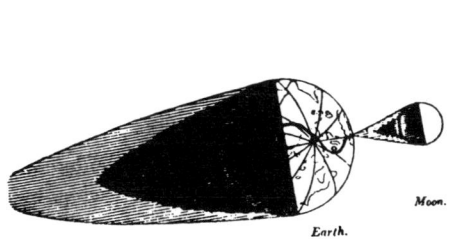
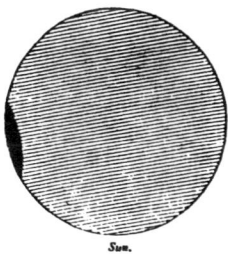

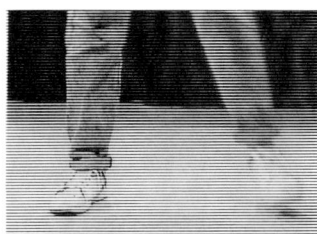

'WAXING & WANING INFLUENCES'

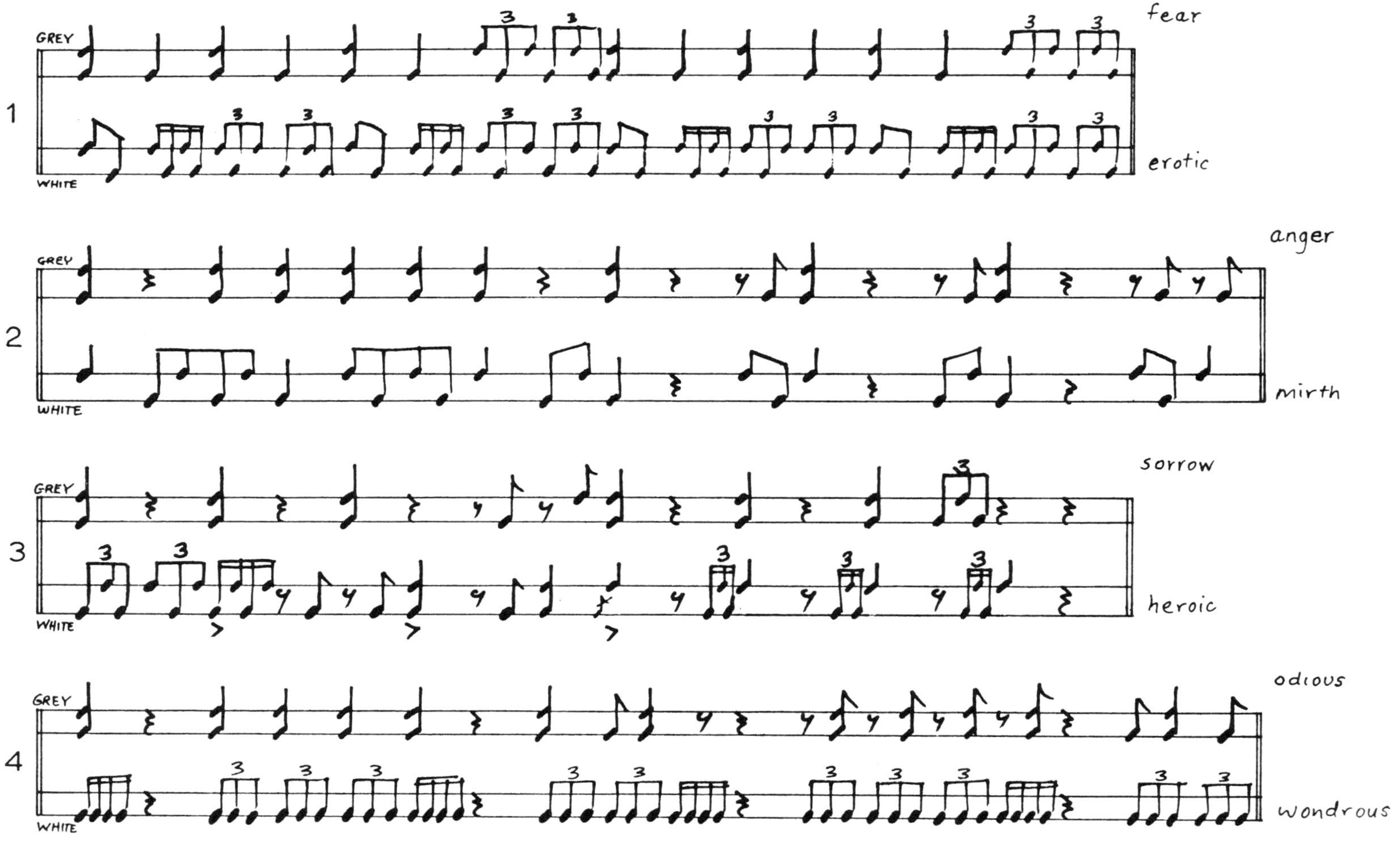

THE FOUR PHASES.

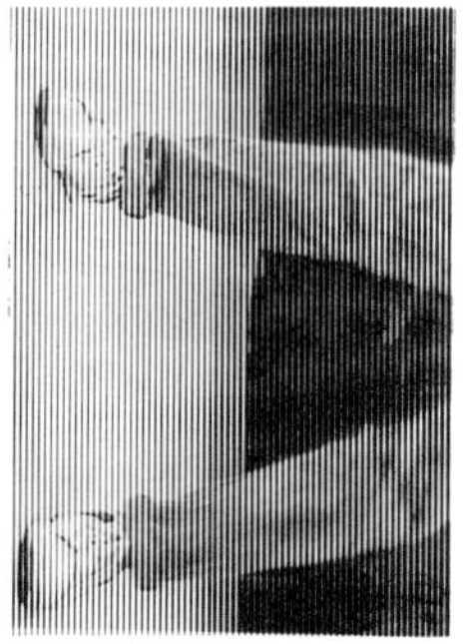

transformation can begin at either end of the grey rhythm. One beat of the grey is exploded into white for every cycle of the grey rhythm. Both sounded and silent beats of the grey matrix are used for the development of the white rhythms, which are usually more complex than their grey equivalents. For example, a triplet might replace a crotchet on one cycle. This process of replacement continues until the total white rhythm is blasted from the grey.

Waxing Influence: During the first waxing stage of the piece, only one drummer will remain on the rhythm with which she began. She may or may not be using the same sound source with which she began. The other drummers will leave their rhythm, seeking and joining at the same stage of development as the rhythm they left, the dominant waxing rhythm. The peak of a waxing influence occurs when all four drummers are playing one rhythm, not necessarily in unison, to the same pulse and on the same sound source. The idea that gives the essential dynamic to the waxing influence is that drummers must remain open to influence, ready to change from the sound source and the rhythm they are playing to what they regard is, or will be, the dominant influence. Progress toward the peaking influence may be marked by any of the characteristics that occur in any human group moving to a common goal. They may range between, and include, the two extremes of obsequience, where a drummer may give immediate allegiance to another drummer's rhythm and/or sound source, and recalcitrance, where a drummer holds out on her own rhythm and/or sound source against the dominant sound and rhythm until the last moment. Every drummer must finally join the dominant influence, however, with one exception (see under "Revolutionary Soloist").

Example: The four drummers begin on four separate grey rhythms. One player might begin abstracting to black. The other three might be developing their whites. At some point, the black drummer will be aware that white rhythms rather than black are dominant. She might decide to pursue black in the hope that someone will come across to her influence, but it is likely, because of her obvious minority, that she will go across to one of the white rhythms being played. Two people will then be playing the same white rhythm, though not necessarily in unison. The black drummer will have picked up her new white rhythm at about the same stage she had reached with her black; i.e., if she was halfway through her black, she will pick up the white development at the same stage. The other two drummers playing separate white rhythms will become aware that they are now each in a minority position. Either one of them will join the other two, so that three drummers are playing the same rhythm, and the dominant position of that rhythm is assured, or instead of joining the other two, she may link up with the rhythm being played by the other minority drummer, achieving a balance with two sets of two drummers each playing a separate white rhythm. One drummer from either group must then break rank and go over to the other group, assuring the dominance of its rhythm. The group moves over to a single sound source by a similar method of remaining open to influence. The change, say, from drum to metal, need not be abrupt. When changing, the drummer may begin on drum, move to playing both metal and drum, and then phase out the drum, ending by playing entirely on metal.

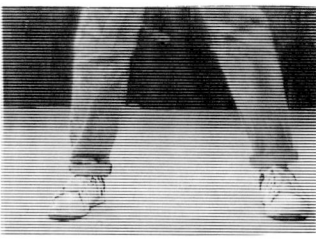

Obviously, this example is only one of many possible combinations. Each should be worked out under the idea that from disparate beginnings an influence will make itself felt and will gather force until it dominates, peaks, and inevitably begins to wane.

Looping: When an influence is peaking and every drummer is playing the same rhythm on one sound source, any drummer can take a rhythmic loop out from, and back into, the peaking influence. This loop will keep within the phase of the

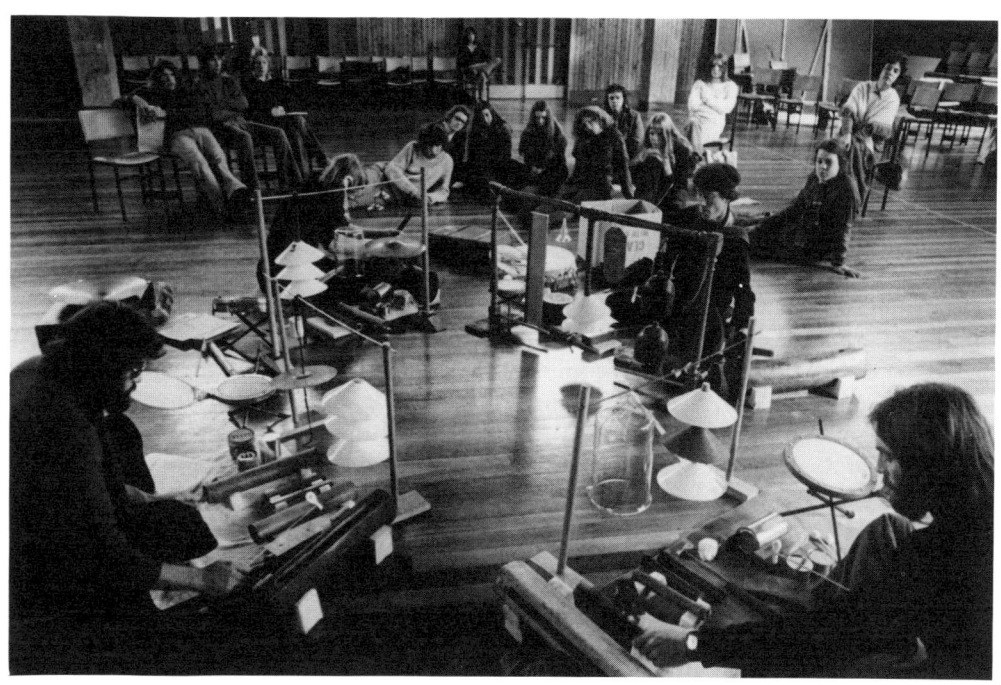

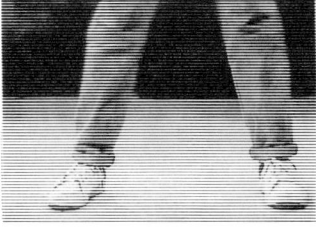

rhythm being played but will be at the opposite pole to that rhythm, coming back through the grey to rejoin the peaking influence. For example, if the group is peaking on a black, the loop would depart into a portion or all of the white rhythm within the same phase and come back through the grey to the black. It would last for only one cycle. Looping can take place before any waning influence starts, but is to be seen as the first indication of decay in a peaking influence and precursor of a waning influence.

Waning Influence: Once an influence is dominant and peaks, it naturally passes into its waning stage. While three drummers are playing the peak, the fourth might do a loop and go back to a grey of the same phase, or simply disregard looping and go straight to the grey. Once on grey, the drummer can, after a time, begin to experiment with all the sound sources again and move finally onto the grey rhythm of another phase. She will be followed out by the other drummers, in their own time. All must pass out through the grey of the phase in which they have just been peaking, then on to another grey and the liberty of experimentation with the sound sources. They are now at a stage identical to the start. The trough follows and a search is underway for the new waxing influence of sound and rhythm.

Tempo: All drummers make a synchronized start on a common pulse. Black rhythms are slower than grey; white rhythms faster than grey. As the progressions away from grey develop, there are therefore two major alternatives:

1. The drummers can keep the common pulse regardless, whether they are developing black or white rhythms. If the waxing influence is white, they will all be developing a faster pulse as they near the peak. If the waxing influence is black, they will all be slowing the common pulse as they approach peak.

2. As drummers move respectively into their black or white rhythms, they progressively adjust their individual speeds to suit the rhythm. In the trough between peaks, where no one influence is dominant, some drummers may then be slightly slowing the pulse, others speeding it, and the common pulse will disintegrate. As the waxing influence gathers way, all drummers will regain the common pulse. Peaking occurs on a common pulse; looping usually does, and the common pulse is maintained during the waning influence.

Ending: The drummer who finds herself leading a black peak may find she has abstracted into silence while the other players are still moving toward the peak. She should remain silent, then control the peak by looping out before all the other drummers have reached silence. If all players do fall silent, the piece ends. This fall over the black peak into silence is the means to deliberately end the piece.

Revolutionary Soloist: If a player feels a particular waxing influence unsuited to her needs, but recognizes also that the influence has reached the point where it will be the dominant waxing influence, she may attempt to draw the other players away. Initially she will draw attention to herself by using any or all of the sound sources, freely exploiting them, but will finish by concentrating on a single sound source different from the sound source still waxing behind her, and on a single rhythm selected from any of the rhythms within the four phases, with the exception of the rhythm still waxing behind her. At this point the other drummers will decide if they will go over to the newly suggested influence. If they continue with the waxing influence they were playing before the advent of the soloist, the soloist must

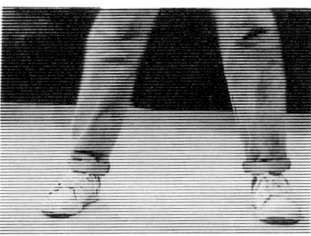

fall back to their waxing influence or fall silent. If the players decide to go over to the soloist's new suggested influence, they should go over quickly, and the soloist's suggested influence then becomes the new waxing influence.

Like life, the piece can reflect a gamut of emotions and likewise a desire at times to obliterate certain ones. Any objections to sounds or behavior might be channeled through the revolutionary solo, and words and gestures are as valid as music. In fact, verbal honesty could result in direct response from players (and/or audience)—a new waxing influence.

Note: Players might exaggerate black or white roles as they see fit.
Geoff Chapple and Philip Dadson, '74

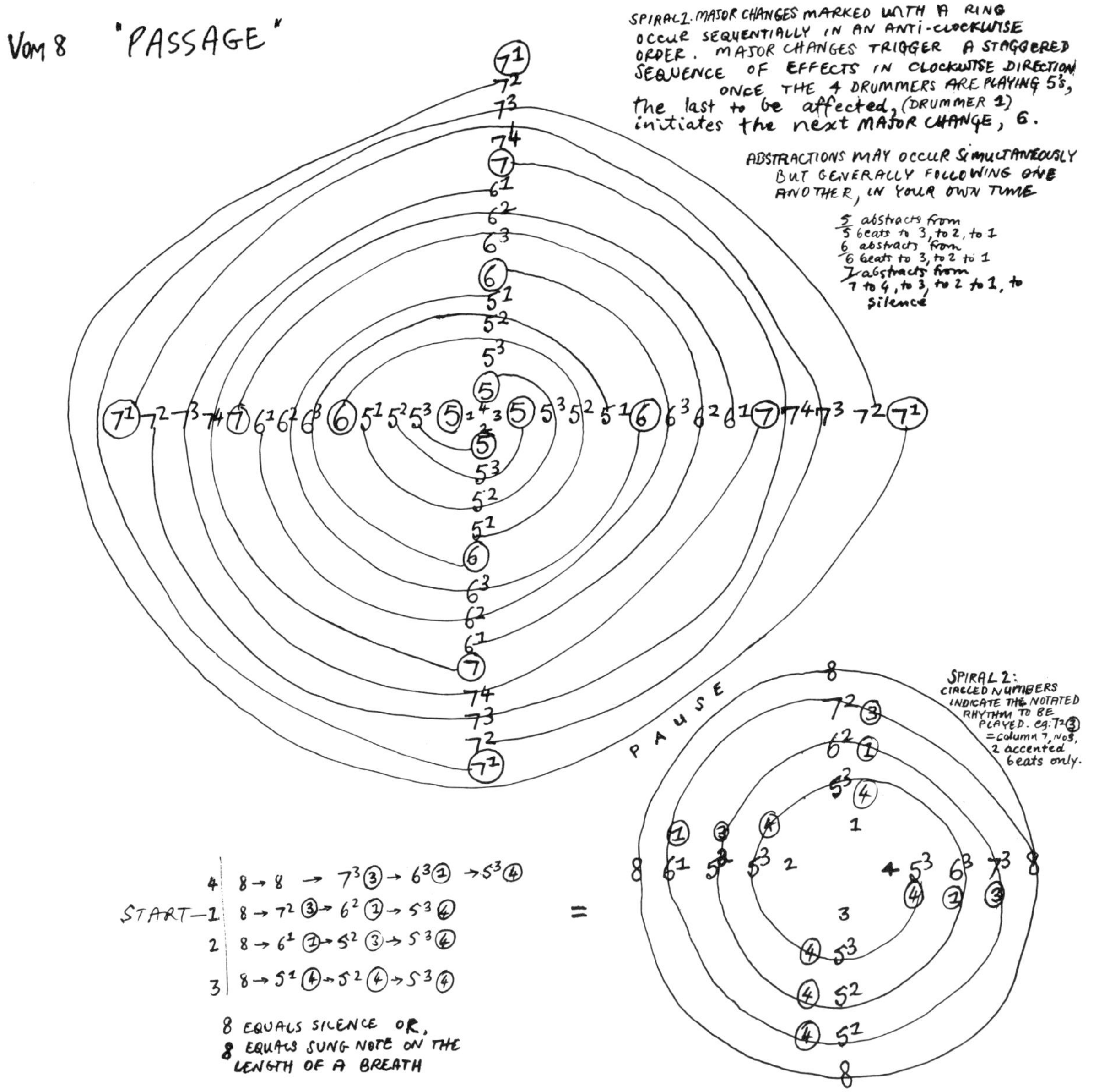

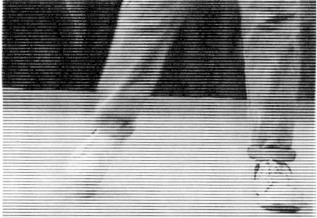

8. Passage
   Part 1:

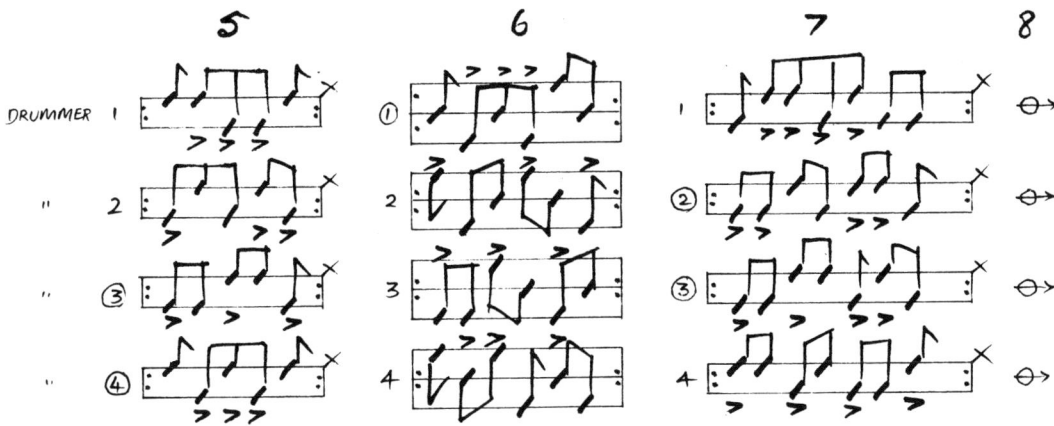

Part 2:

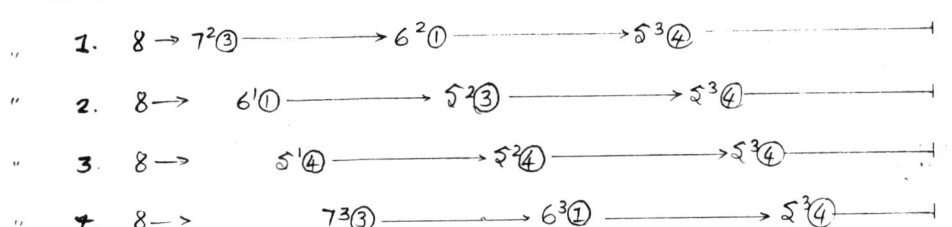

Passage Notes: The four drummers sit in a circle facing each other. Each has an array of randomly pitched sound sources: skin, metal, glass, wood, plastic, stone, bone, matching categories of resonantly short to long, harmonically simple to complex, and aurally deep to high. *art, 58*

Rhythms: Patterns 5 have two or more sources of short resonance, one high and one low, 6, three or more of medium resonance, high, middle, and low; and 7, two or more of long resonance, medium and low.

Fives and 7s are played on two sources, and 6s on three. The sign X above a repeat sign indicates that the sound sources are alternated each repetition. For example:

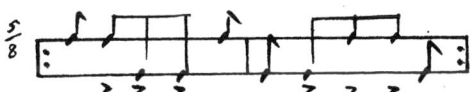

This also occurs in 6 once the pattern is abstracted to 3 beats.
   Rhythm abstractions are as follows:
      5s from 5 beats, to 3 accented, to 2, to 1
      6s from 6, to 3, to 2, to 1
      7s from 7, to 4, to 3, to 2, to 1

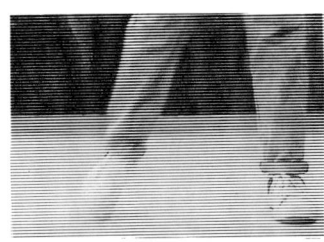

Procedure: The piece is in 3 parts. One, which corresponds to spiral 1; two, the pause between (sung notes on the length of a breath); and three, spiral 2.

The general procedure in part 1 is one of cause and staggered effects. Entries, and all subsequent changes, are sequential. Each new full rhythm (a major change) triggers abstractions by the other players (see diagram).

Part 1 begins at 5 and proceeds through to 7; 8 equals a hiatus into which drummers abstract out of 7 and sing a drone note on the length of a breath.

Part 2 returns to 5. Players one by one leave off the sung note and resume drumming. The overall sound is sparse to begin and dense to end. It begins very slowly and gradually accelerates to the 5s, which are played dissynchronously; and after a time ends abruptly.

The entire process in parts 1 and 2 should be gradual, allowing time for composite patterns to emerge. Sound sources are selected in accord with the overall sound, and once selected remain constant for each rhythm through full and abstracted patterns.

Option: Instructions for Two Reed Players (e.g., soprano sax and oboe), producing beats and overtones whenever possible.

Soprano aligns to Drummer 1 (can play rhythmic patterns of either Drummer 1 or 2). Oboe aligns to Drummer 4 (can play rhythmic patterns of either Drummer 3 or 4). Both winds follow an identical procedure pattern.

Drummer 1	*Wind 1*
5 full	Portamento up to 5th from tonic (of choice) and sustain
5 (3)	Full rhythms in octaves
5 (2)	5 (3)
5 (1)	5 (2)
6 full	5 (1)
6 (3)	6 full—6th from tonic in octaves, plus tonic as middle line
6 (2)	6 (3)
6 (1)	6 (2)
7 full	6 (1)
7 (4)	7 full—7th from tonic in octaves
7 (3)	7 (4)
7 (2)	7 (3)
7 (1)	7 (2)
Sing 7th of wind	7 (1)
4 singers slur to tonic	tonic—continuous producing of beats when possible
7 (2) very slow	7 (2) continuous tonic counted in cycles of 7 with two references to 7th (= accented beats) each cycle
6 (2)	6 (2) tonic and 6th
5 (3) accelerate	5 (3) tonic and 5th

General speed acceleration and end abruptly.

Philip Dadson, '74

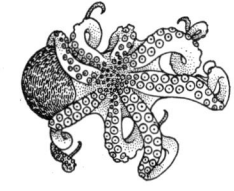

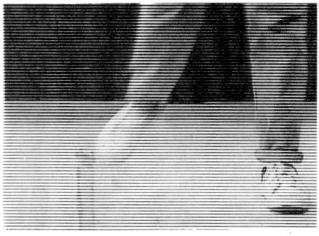

APPENDIX 6
SOME INSTRUMENT IDEAS

There's nothing quite as exciting as building a homemade instrument and using it for making your own music.

The physical world is one huge resource for percussion players. While the industry trend is toward ever-increasisng electronic and computer sophistication and minituarization, ours has been toward natural acoustics and often large sculptural constructions with natural and industrial materials. The most developed of these is the tuned percussion "stations," giant pan-pipe-styled racks. Each station (high, medium, and low) has four tiers of

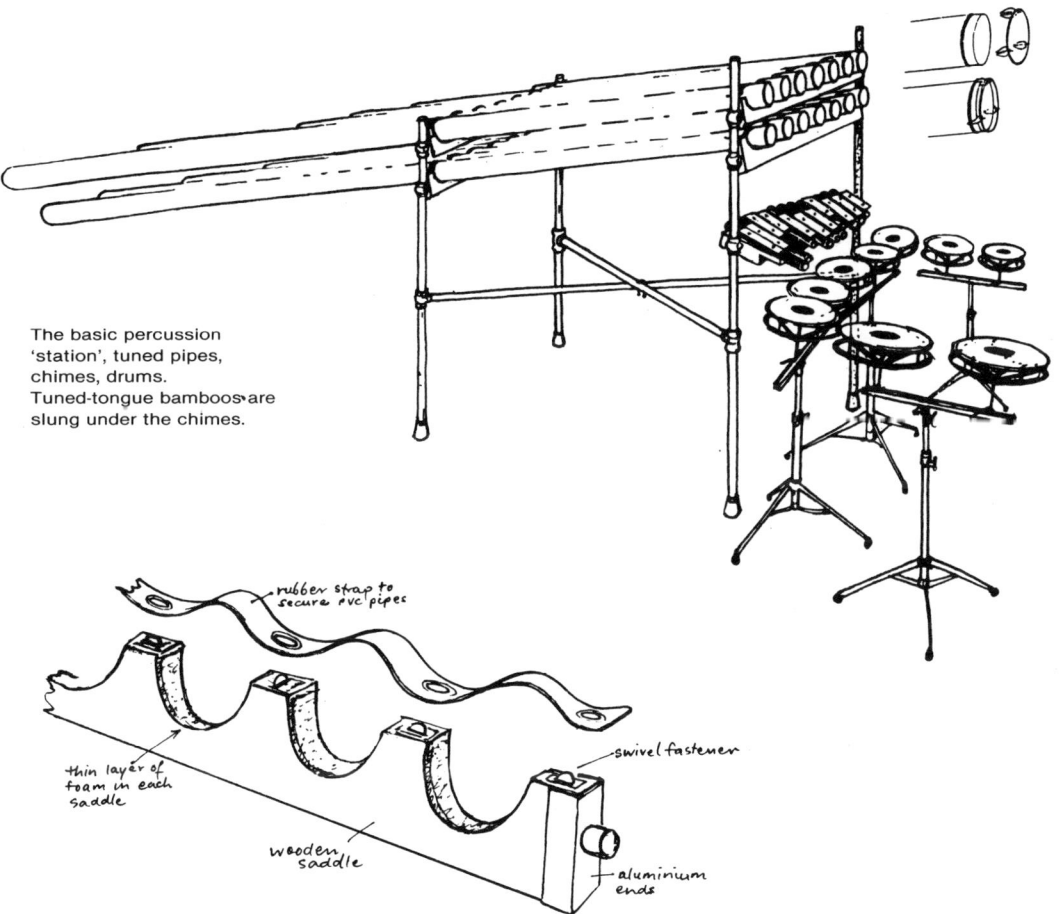

The basic percussion 'station', tuned pipes, chimes, drums. Tuned-tongue bamboos are slung under the chimes.

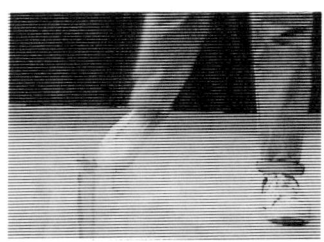

distinct sound sources: 14 end-struck PVC pipes, 14 to 20 tuned chimes, 6 to 8 tuned-tongue bamboos, and 6 to 8 tuned drums (plastic, metal, wood, and skin).

Each player stands at a station, with all the sound sources arranged in front and to either side, like a big switchboard. The pitches in each tier are arranged low to high, left to right.

Each station, with its easily accessible and different tonal layers—PVC pipes, metal chimes, bamboos, and drums—ideally permits the exchange of any one tuned source for another. Rhythmic/melodic lines are enriched by this potential, where a type of hocketing can be acheved by one player. Two or more stations in combination can produce an intricate hocket texture (e.g.; through the 7 sections of "Gung Ho 1, 2, 3D").

To get different combinations of sounds, the player has to make different shapes in space. As the repeating rhythmic patterns swing from high to low and back again, each player sets up a kind of rhythmic semaphore that's just as much a part of a piece as the sound is—and playing this instrument keeps you fit!

Inventory of Pipe Sizes and Lengths Used in the From Scratch High, Medium, and Low "Percussion Stations"

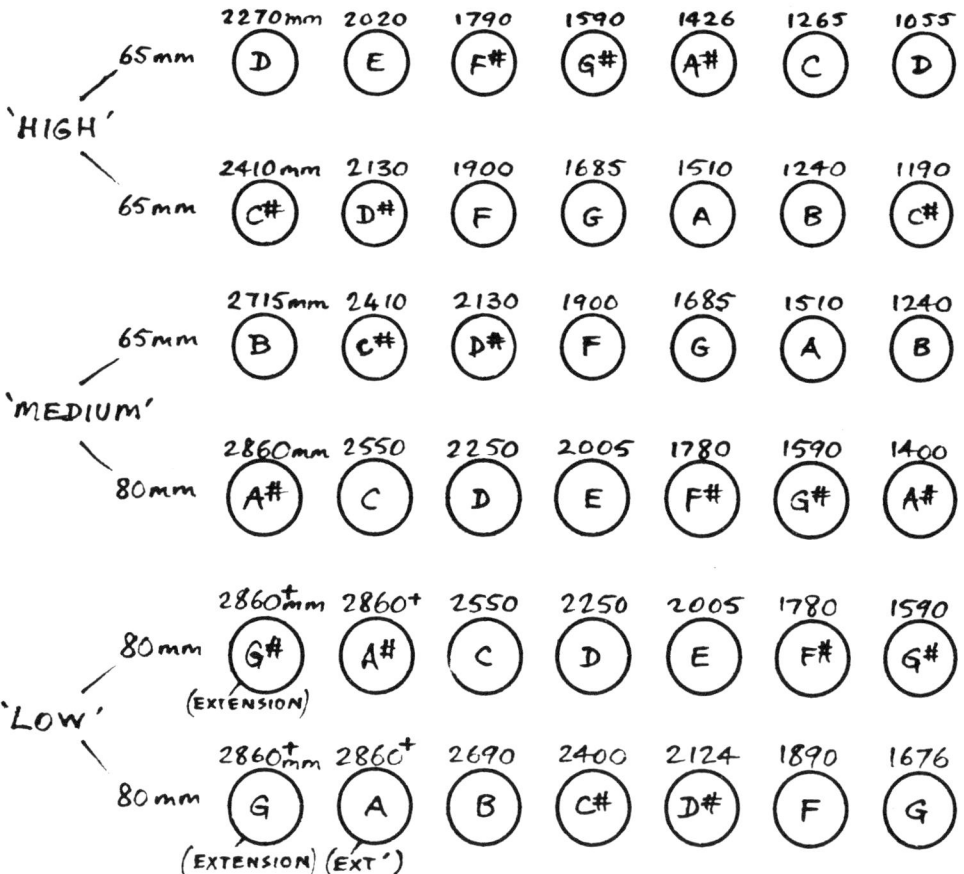

'HIGH'

65mm: 2270mm D, 2020 E, 1790 F#, 1590 G#, 1426 A#, 1265 C, 1055 D

65mm: 2410mm C#, 2130 D#, 1900 F, 1685 G, 1510 A, 1240 B, 1190 C#

'MEDIUM'

65mm: 2715mm B, 2410 C#, 2130 D#, 1900 F, 1685 G, 1510 A, 1240 B

80mm: 2860mm A#, 2550 C, 2250 D, 2005 E, 1780 F#, 1590 G#, 1400 A#

'LOW'

80mm: 2860+mm G# (extension), 2860+ A#, 2550 C, 2250 D, 2005 E, 1780 F#, 1590 G#

80mm: 2860+mm G (extension), 2860+ A (ext'), 2690 B, 2400 C#, 2124 D#, 1890 F, 1676 G

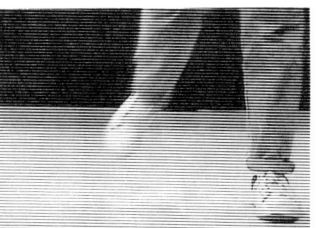

(Note: The previous lengths are not exact for 12-tone equal temperament. Adjustable sleeves are necessary for fine-tuning purposes. On the low station, 3 extension pipes are required for low G, G#, and A. G#, for example, has an extension pipe 590 mm, plus sleeve.)

PVC pipe expands and contracts with changes in temperature; therefore the lengths in the inventory illustration are for the hot extreme. To allow for all conditions, a tuning sleeve is fitted to each length (externally or internally), and tuning of pipes is done prior to any performance. We learned this the hard way in Papua New Guinea (Sth Pacific Fest' Arts 1980), where the heat raised the tuning of the pipes a good semi-tone.

For the 65-mm pipes we use "outer" adjustable sleeves approximately 120 mm long. These were made by heating (dry heat or boiling water) one section of pipe and forcing it over another of the same diameter. (There is a heating point at which the PVC will expand without collapsing). Some fine sanding is necessary to get a snug sliding fit.

For the 80-mm pipes we use an "inner" adjustable sleeve approximately 200 mm long. In New Zealand there were two main producers of PVC pipes. Selected lengths of one brand fitted snugly inside the other, presenting the solution for a tuning sleeve.

You will need to experiment a bit to get inserts that are a good fit yet movable. We use a heavy-duty white gaffer tape (used in the film industry) to position off the sleeves once tuned. A small rectangle on the underside is adequate.

For notes beyond the manufactured length (e.g., the bottom 4 notes of the "low" station, and any extra set-up of very low notes), we use extension pipes with joining rings, and adjustable sleeves in the ends.

Tuning sleeves, besides providing for fine tuning, give the instruments a tuning flexibility that allows for systems other than 12-tone equal.

In addition to playing the pipes with open ends, we use a membrane on the end of the pipes to both change the tone and allow the use of mallets. The sound and tone are quite different from open pipes.

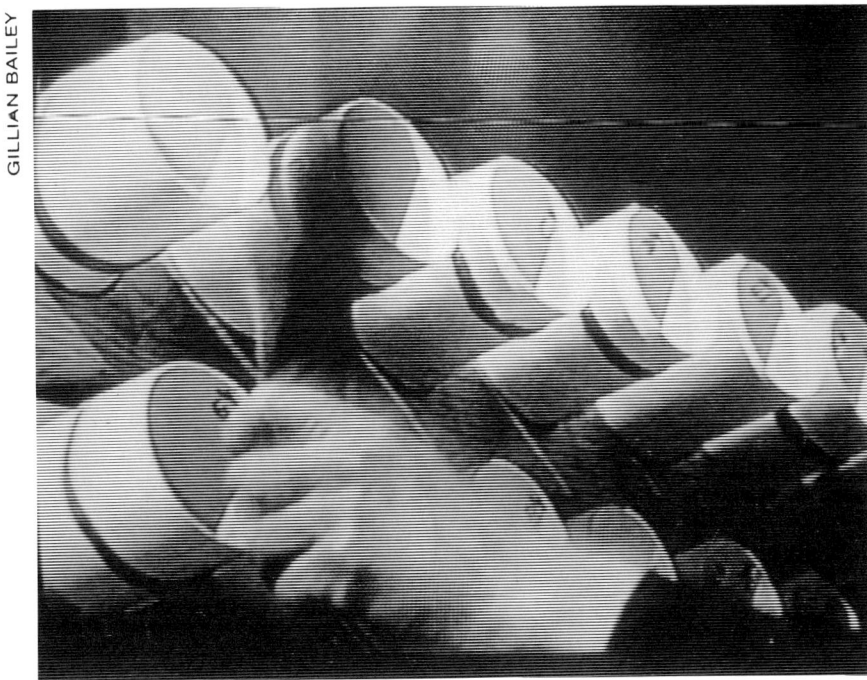

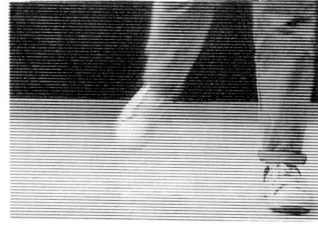

At first, we used plastic cups, which give an interesting but indefinite-pitched tone. Later, we improved this by using a high-strength flexible plastic (lexan). A disc is attached to each pipe with an air space between. A more recent instrument, the "eye-drum" stations, use 1 mm-thick clear PVC.

Bats for Striking PVC Pipes

We use a rubber lamination, the same used for sandals or thongs. There are a variety of these and you need to find a lamination about 20 mm thick with a hard wearing surface on one side. Usually, when cut to size, the two sides will produce different sounds. The harder side has more punch and slap combined with the tube tone, and the softer side is more mellow.

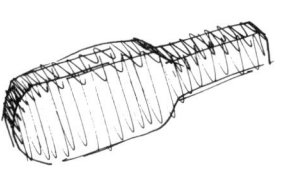 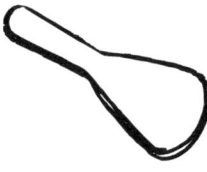 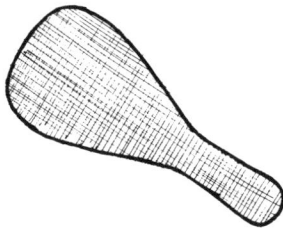

Make sure the strike area is big enough to cover the size of pipe you are using.

For the hand-held smaller diameter tube bundles, we use a softer rubber. It's very expensive but worth it for the sound. There is virtually no slap, which is important with the smaller diameter pipes where the tone is not as full.

Hand-held PVC

There is a big range of grey PVC plumbing and electrical pipe available on the market, ranging from 20 mm in diameter to 120 mm plus. We use a plumbing variety of diameters 40 to 50 mm for hand-held percussion.

A number of tuned lengths, both open at both ends and closed one end, are fixed together in threes mainly, and end-struck with a soft rubber bat. This way you can produce interesting chords of sound.

A pipe closed at one end will produce the same note as an open pipe twice its length. There is a slight difference of tone. Short lengths with one closed end are not very satisfactory, i.e., anything less than 500 mm long (diameter 40–50 mm) produces more contact sound than tone.

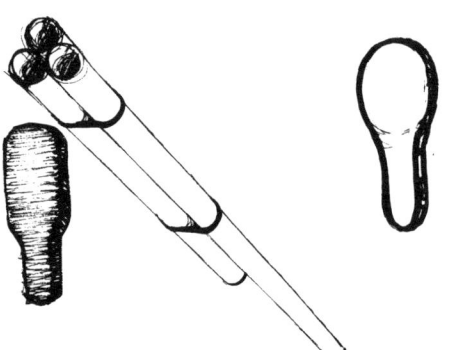

WARNING: PVC is a toxic material. Avoid inhaling fumes and dust particles. Use adequate ventilation when cutting or heating etc.

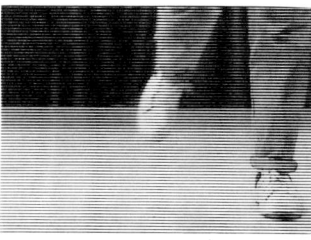

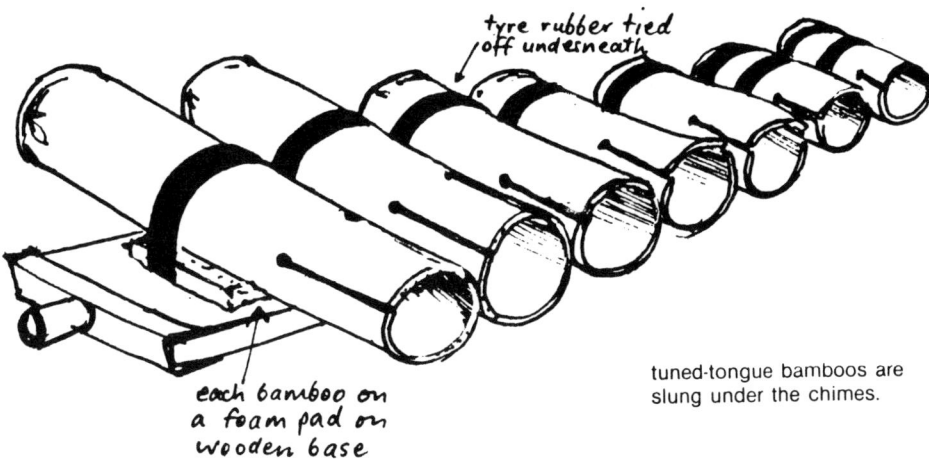

each bamboo on a foam pad on wooden base

tyre rubber tied off underneath

tuned-tongue bamboos are slung under the chimes.

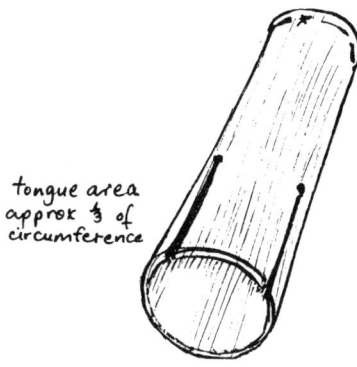

tongue area approx ⅓ of circumference

Tuned-tongue Bamboos

These were inspired from reading about the BOOs—an instrument devised by American composer/inventor Harry Partch and based on the tuned-tongue principle (matching a vibrating tongue to a resonator) as used in some parts of S.E. Asia and Africa (the Mbira, or thumb piano, for example). We wanted a warm wood tone to add to the PVC, metal, and drum combination, so when some large-size dry bamboo came our way, tuned-tongue bamboos were the result.

If you can get good-quality large-size bamboo, the results are rewarding. The tone is clear, short, dry but mellow.

Making the tongue involves cutting a slot into the open end of a bamboo tube, with or without a closed end. Both will work, but a tube open at both ends will be twice the length of one closed at one end, if both are the same pitch. The other end of the tongue works as a resonator. The tongue end has a slot cut into it—two parallel cuts on the top face of the tube. Tuning involves cutting the slot until the tongue end resonates with the cavity. Because bamboo is of variable thickness and diameter, no two bamboos are exactly alike; i.e., two bamboos tuned to the same pitch may be of slightly different lengths and have slightly different length slots. In general, though, slots are from 1/3 (lowest tones) to approximately 1/2 (middle and high tones) the tube length.

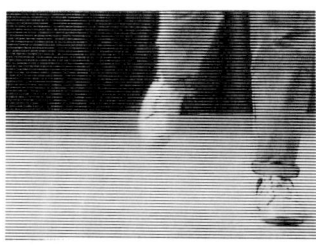

Pitching a length takes practice, but the general idea is that the starting pitch of the tube (end-blown or struck) will be raised a 4th to a 5th when the tongue is perfectly coupled to the resonator. This is tested by blowing into one of the slots. If the blow tone (edge-tone) is slightly lower than the tongue, then the best match is achieved.

One easy way to cut the slots in the bamboo is to first mark the size of the tongue with two parallel lines on the outside of the bamboo. At a point on both lines, just less than 1/3 the length of the tube (this is for tubes closed at one end with a node or wooden plug), drill a hole the width you want the slot to be (4 mm approximately). Using a sharp short blade—the Stanley variety is good—split the bamboo carefully down a line from the open end to the outside edge of the drilled hole. Repeating this down a line to the inside edge of the drilled hole, you can remove a bamboo sliver. Do this on both sides.

Check the pitch of the tongue against the pitch of the cavity by tapping the tongue and blowing across the base of the slot (edge-tone). As you lengthen the slot, the tongue pitch goes down and the cavity pitch goes up. Remember, best coupling is when the two pitches are just short of matching—the blow tone slightly lower. (Thank you, Harry Partch. It works!)

To lengthen the slots, drill or saw (jigsaw) both sides evenly, 1 to 2 mm at a time as it approaches coupling. This stage is very critical and 1 mm too much may deaden the tone. If you go too far, shorten the overall length of the tube and go for the next higher pitch in your series.

If the tongue is too sharp, the bamboo is rasped on top at the base of the tongue. This flattens it. If the tongue is too flat, the end of the tongue is rasped very slightly underneath (thanks again, Harry).

The mounting method we use involves fitting them—low to high, left to right—onto a wooden base, with foam pads between the base and the bamboos. Each bamboo is fastened with a strip of rubber cut from a car tire's inner tube. The rubber encircles the bamboo, passing through slots at each side of the tube, and is tied underneath the base.

Each base supporting 7 or 8 tubes is mounted on the stations underneath the metal chimes with the tongue ends protruding. The tongue is struck on the open end with soft or medium mallets.

Tuned Chimes and Gongs

We use several different styles of chimes and gongs, all made from tube and sheet aluminium. When selecting material, make sure there are no obvious imperfections such as extrusion ridges, as this can be detrimental to the tone.

Tuned-tongue chimes

Both round and square section aluminum tube can be used, though square is both easier to mill and gives a flat playing surface. The making technique for each individual chime is virtually the same as for a tuned-tongue bamboo, in that the two ends of a tube length, slotted and resonator, are matched to reinforce one another. The resonator end, however, can be open—for medium to high notes—or closed off (with a rubber or cork plug) for the longer medium-to-low notes. I use a 40-mm square tube. It's a good chunky size and is good both mounted and hand-held. Cutting the slot is easiest done on a milling machine where you can mill the slot dead center down two opposite faces of the tube.

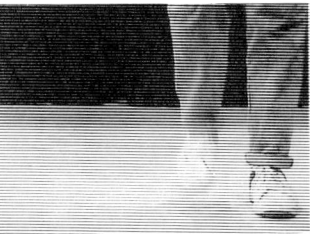

To get started, cut a trial length of tube 42 cm long. Mark a center line down two opposite sides and cut a slot exactly 144 mm down each side (hacksaw or milling machine). Although the resonator end is not correctly matched, the slotted end (looking a bit like a tuning fork) should produce the note of D-natural one octave above mid-C. Now, by trimming the resonator end so that the edge-tone (checked by blowing across the base of the slot) is slightly lower than the tongue end, a match will be achieved to produce full resonance. You should end up with a length of tube approximately 393 mm long, open at both ends. Now get a bucket of water and immerse the resonator end of the tube into the water, all the while striking the slotted end on one of the non-slotted faces. You will discover an alternative closed position where resonance occurs. This demonstrates the alternative method where a plug can be inserted and the resonator end effectively shortened, and the surplus cut off.

Round section chimes

Hand-held bells can easily be made from cut lengths of round aluminum tube, lightly fastened or held at the central node. The lengths can get quite long but look good when arranged in sets of tuned lengths as hand-held instruments.

Gongs

Try making gongs by cutting circular and triangular shapes from sheet aluminum. The thinner the gauge, the lower the pitch range; the thicker, the higher. Gongs such as these are tuned by carefully hammering a center "dimple," which affects the range by up to a fifth from the untuned state (hence dimple gongs).

To find suspension points, lay the gong flat on small foam blocks and sprinkle the gong surface with fine sand or salt. Gently strike the gong in the center and the salt or sand grains will form into a nodal ring, where holes can be drilled without affecting gong pitch or resonance.

Spun Acoustic Drones

Spun acoustic drones have been an integral part of *From Scratch* music since the mid-70s as both visual and sound accompaniment to the percussion. Common to all is the acoustic principle of whirling to produce continuous sound either by vibration and/or air pressure. In performance the instruments dramatically stress the circular and repetitive shapes of the music.

The best known and most elementary of the spun sound makers is the "bullroarer," an instrument common to many tribal situations. A version more familiar to children is made by spinning a short wooden or plastic ruler around on the end of a looped cord.

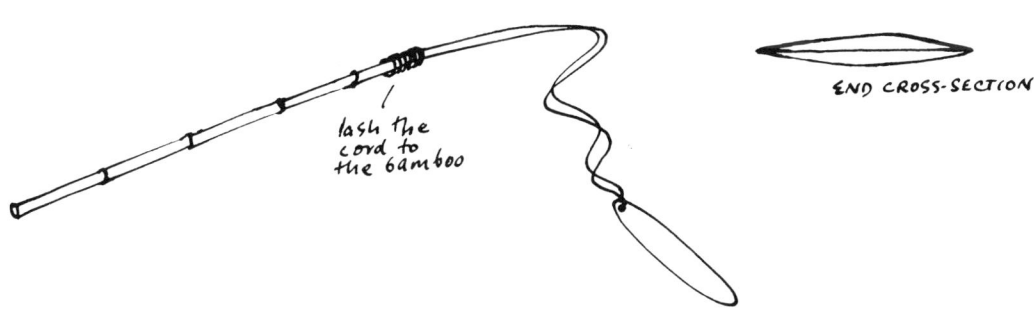

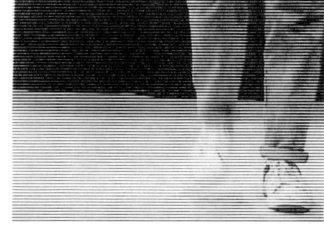

A more effective one can be made by using thin plywood cut to an elongated oval shape 30 to 50 cm long. Shape the ply at the edges for aerodynamics and attach a 1m to 2m long looped cord to one end of the instrument. Attach the other end to a flexible but solid bamboo handle.

On one "Solar Plexus" occasion, we used a large number of these and other spun drones (including speakers and portable amps) in Maungawhau crater as part of the dawn-to-dusk winter solstice drumming event. En masse, they make a very impressive sound.

Different in principle to the bullroarer is the "growler," which transmits vibrations along a nylon line from a point of friction to a membrane and resonator.

The growler (a drum membrane) and the "whizzer," (a cymbal) are blow-ups of a smaller idea, a Chinese children's toy, which when spun produces an insect-like buzzing.

A nylon loop spinning around a rosined section of wooden handle creates friction that is passed down the taut nylon line as vibration, to a membrance receiver—such as a drumskin—which in turn amplifies the sound. Small tambourines are ideal, although the shell of the drum may need weighting with plastercine to stop wobble. These are spun around the head to produce a roughly pitched continuous sound. (Used en masse at the end of "Drumwheel" Part 2, 1979.)

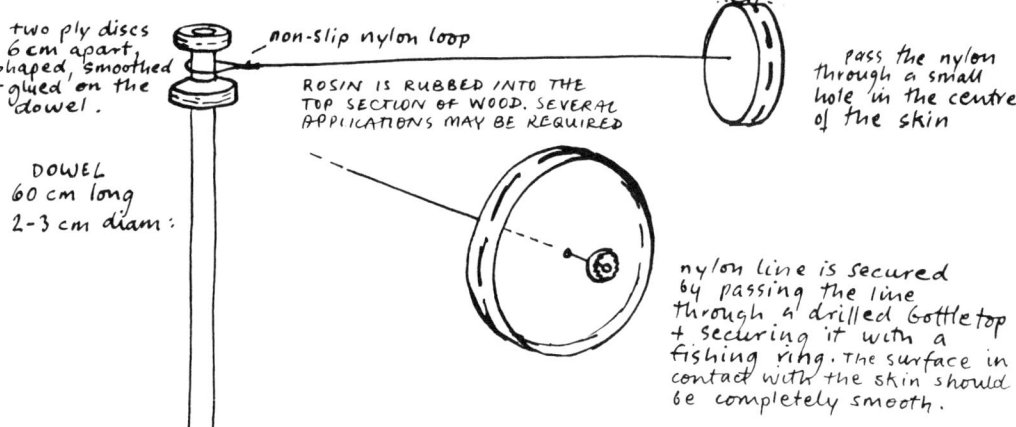

A variation on the growler is to use a short length of 80-mm PVC downpipe with a plastic cup secured on one end. The length of the pipe affects the relative pitch of the sound.

Like the drum growler, the nylon passes through the center of the plastic cup, then through a washer of a smooth, strong material—nylon, metal—and is lastly secured by a fishing ring. The cup can be either contact glued or secured by a ring of PVC cut from a joiner sleeve. A number of these at different lengths can produce an interesting sound texture, especially outdoors.

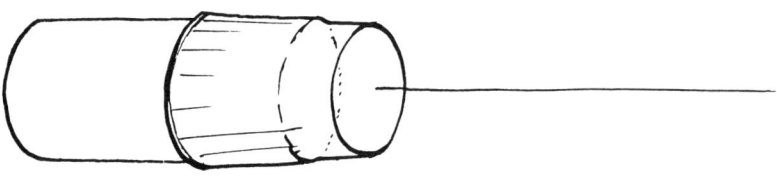

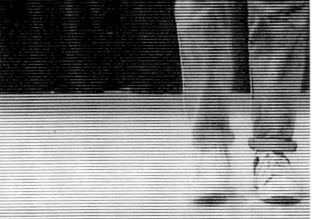

Using the same principle, try small cymbals or discs of thin aluminum spun on the nylon line.

The major thing to consider with these spun drones is safety. Be sure the nylon is strong enough and that all the knots and loops are thoroughly secure.

A gentle drone, by contrast, is produced by singing a constant pitched note into one end of a flexible rubber or plastic hose, and spinning the other end around above your head at the same time. A meter-length or longer of flexible hosing is good.

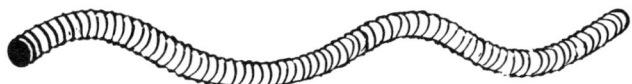

We call this a "hummer." Like any kind of pipe, length affects pitch and the best result is had by matching the pipe length to the note required. Somewhat similar to this is the "trom" tube. We use both flexible and rigid thin-walled polythene and PVC pipes for this one. The playing technique requires an embouchure similar to that for a trombone and other brass, and we learned a rotation breathing technique to obtain continuous, constant pitched sound. The flexible pipe is spun around the head while blowing (similar to the hummer) and with the rigid pipe we turned slowly around on the spot while playing.

The "warbler" is also a flexible hose but of a special kind. It is a thin-walled plastic hose with a corrugated wall, used commercially for both plumbing and "sound-toy" uses. Cut to length and spun with varying speeds, the pipe produces a pure sequence of harmonics.

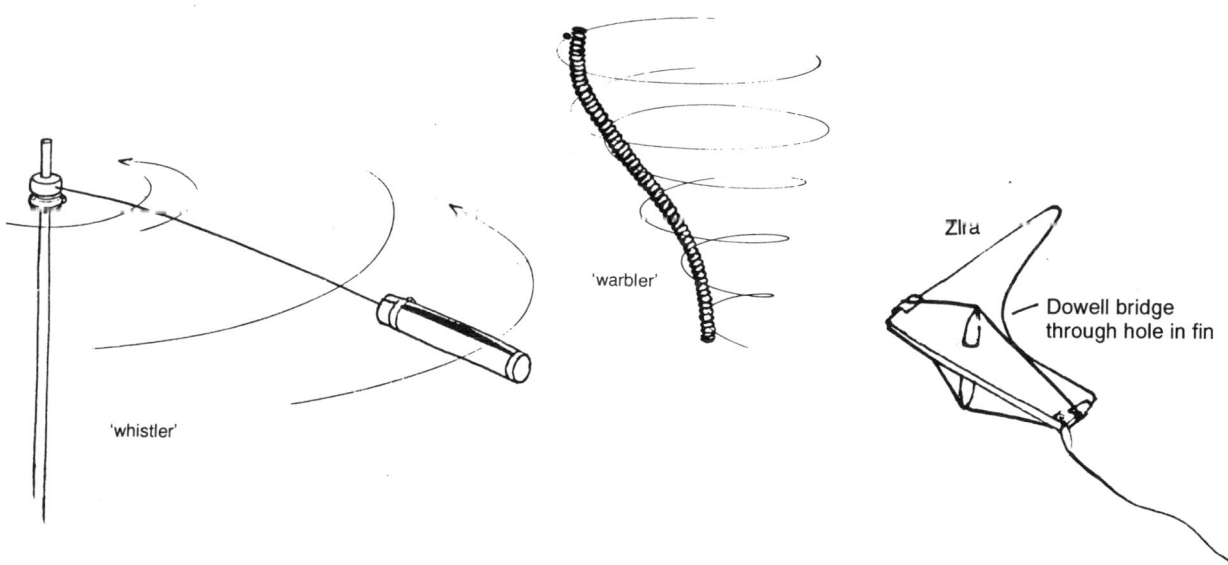

The "whistler" is based on another child's toy, a small tin tube with a slot, which when spun on a string, produces a bird-like whistle. Our whistlers used tin cylinders from 400 to 500 mm long. A tin cap is soldered into both ends and a plumbing ring is used to tune the slot. The cylinder is spun by connecting it to a metal rod approximately 1 m long. The other end of the rod is connected to a waxed wooden ring and is spun around a long dowel rod at least 230 mm in diameter.

Where a regular fixed pitch is required, the whistler would have to be the most temperamental of all the spun sources.

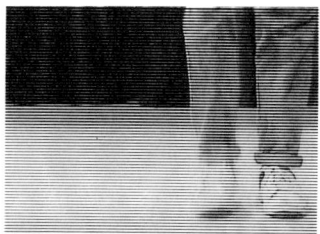

The most recent of the spun devices is the "Jilzira," based on a small instrument called the "zira," used by Australian artist Jill Scott. The zira is a small boomerang-shaped ply sound board with a bridge on each side and a rubber band stretched around. When spun, the band vibrates and is amplified through the sound board. The small version produces a high-pitched insect-like sound. Our larger versions produce a more vocal-like sound.

I have made them both with and without resonators and have had equal success. With resonator, a length of bamboo with a node at each end was used. The bamboo tube is split down the middle and each half is glued, top and bottom, to the front edge of the sound board. A hole corresponding to the area of bamboo is removed from the ply before gluing. A 50 to 60 mm bridge is fitted to each side of the resonator.

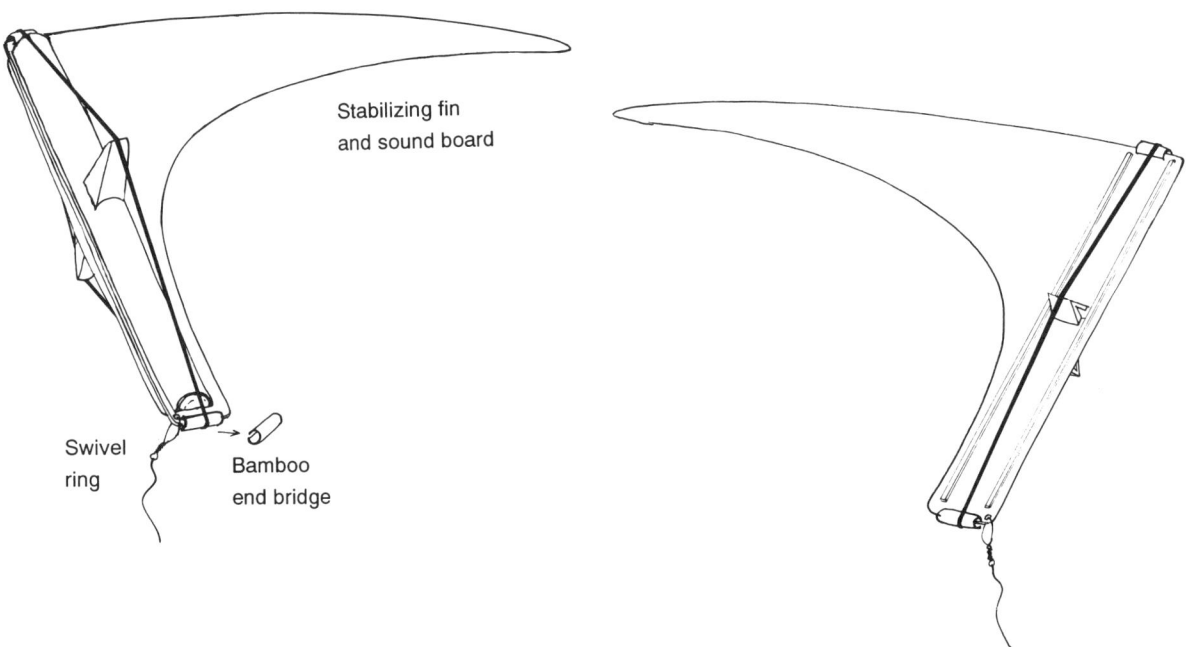

Without resonator, strengthening is required at the front edge to stop the ply's buckling under tension from the rubber band(s). I did this by gluing four wooden strips, two at the front edge, top and bottom, and two 60 to 70 mm in parallel to the front edge. This provides a strip along which the bridges—top and bottom—can be slid for tuning purposes. A large rubber band (as used in post offices for parcels) is stretched around the tips of the two bridges and is tuned to a chord of four notes. When the Jilzira is spun on a long string, the four divisions of band vibrate and a continuous chord of sound results. With care and a measure of luck, the four divisions of band can be tuned. Speed alters the harmony by bringing different harmonics into play.

With all of these spun sources, the doppler effect adds a (rhythmic) pulsing to the sound.

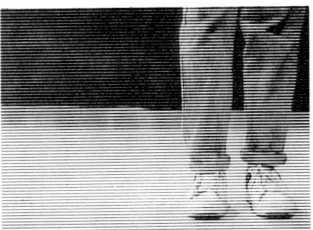

Some Found Sound From Junk and Other Sources
Metal

- Tins of all shapes and sizes—canned food tins, biscuit tins, cake tins, rubbish tins, kerosene tins—with lids on or off, on their sides or upside down on a block of foam. Try also with water inside.
- Try a rubbish bin on blocks of foam rubber with soft beaters.
- Pots, pans, and kettles. Try with and without water.
- Stainless steel basins and old gas tanks make fine gongs.
- Springs of all gauges and sizes. Some long fine springs make good echo reverberators. Akio Suzuki invented an instrument called the "Analapous," which uses long fine springs and cans at each end, a bit like the can and string telephone principle.
- Hubcaps and brake drums—you can get these from car wreckers—are good suspended or mounted on foam.
- Steel, aluminium, and brass pipe—any lengths and diameters.
- When you hold or catch a tube of resonating metal at its exact center—when or after it's been struck—the two ends vibrate equally and produce an upper harmonic. The center node is a still point.
- Acetylene bottle tops. These make good bells if collected in an assortment of sizes and hung from a rack—similarly for brake drums. (For playing at floor level, a simple stand can be made from dowel, wood bases, and a metal rod for the cross bar, from which sound sources can be suspended.)
- Metal discs of thin aluminum, steel, or brass. Hammer a small dish shape into the upper side of the disc to improve resonance and ring.
- Oil drums and oil drum tops. Suspended rims make good gongs. Upended drums are very good and are the source of the Jamaican steel drums.

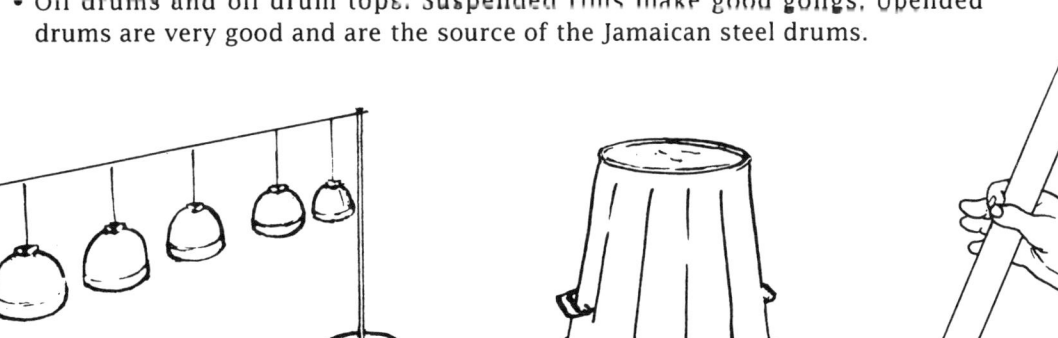

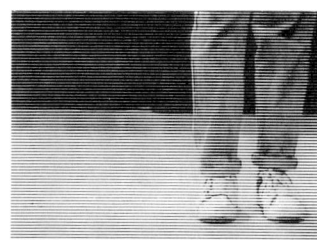

Plastic

- PVC pipes. A variation on the open pipe is to add a plastic cup to one end. Some sizes of plastic cup will fit snugly over the end of a 65- or 80-mm PVC pipe, making a crude membrane that can be finger-tapped or drummed on. Try submerging one end of an open pipe in water, and then tap the other end with a rubber beater. The changing level of water up the pipe will affect the pitch.

- A set of random-tuned or tuned pipes with plastic cups on top can be simply made by strapping/taping the pipes around a central drum of heavy cardboard or industrial pipe.

- Barrels, buckets, and all-sized containers, some of which can make reasonable drums.

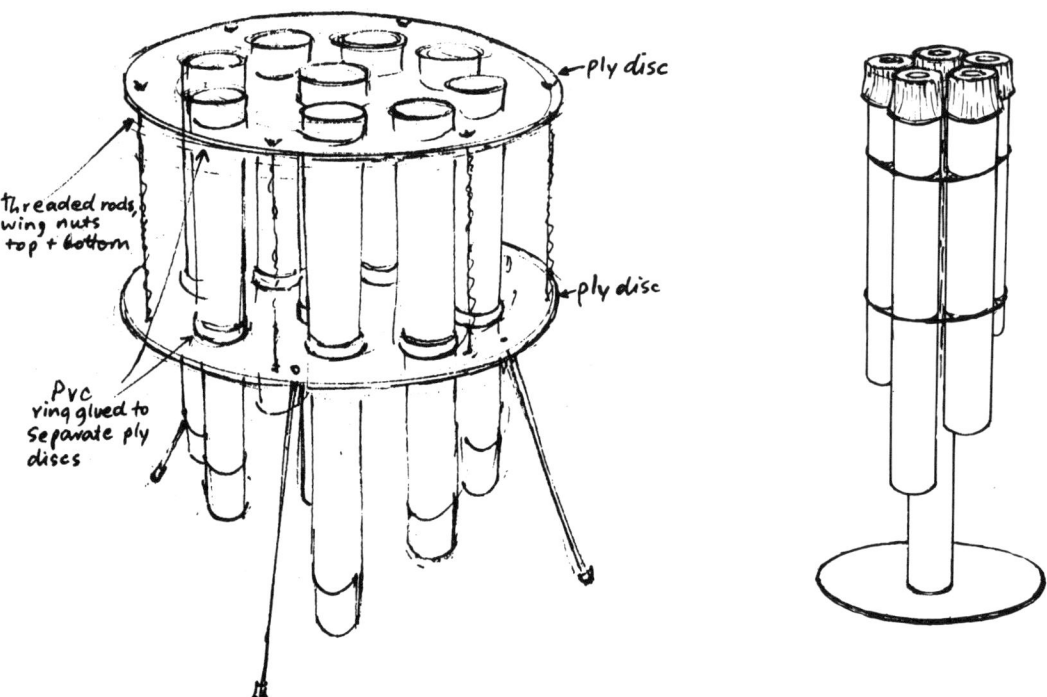

Wood

- Boxes of all sizes, tea chests, and plywood boxes. Plywood nailed onto different-sized box frames make reasonable drums. The ply operates as a crude membrane. Joints should be glued and nailed for best sound.

- Blocks and lengths of dry wood, such as large-size dowel, or cut lengths of dry pine, gum, or hardwoods.

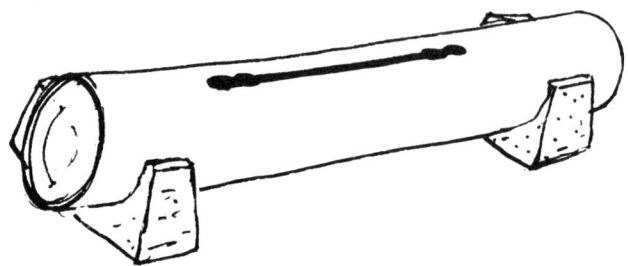

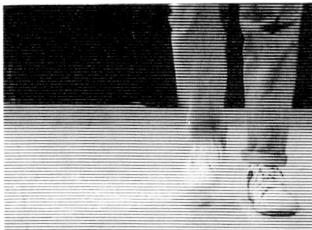

- Short paired lengths make good tuned claves. Longer lengths can be tossed and struck, or suspended or mounted on foam.
- Bamboo (dry), if large sizes, can make quite acceptable slit drums. Cut lengths leaving a node at both ends. Along a line, drill two holes a third of the length in from the ends. Remove the strip between the holes with a sharp blade. Tune the slot to the tube by extending the slot length a drill hole at a time.
- Small and large stamping tubes of bamboo are made by exposing a node at one end and cutting off the other end. The node end is then bounced on a hard surface—earth, asphalt, brick—or, if indoors, on a rubber mat on a hard floor. Similarly you can use PVC pipes with a disc of PVC glued on one end.

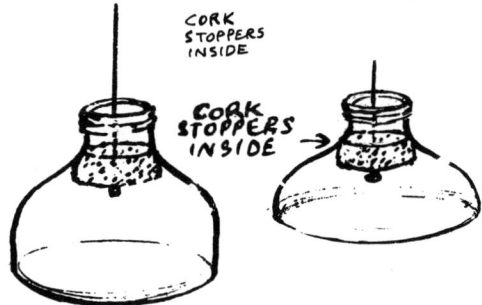

Glass

- Bottles, with and without water. Try a range of types; not all are good. Fill to different levels with water and either arrange in a semi-circle at floor level or suspend from a rack, low to high.
- Half-gallon jars or, better still, acid jars. Remove the jar bottoms at different lengths from the necks (see your local glass cutter). When suspended, they are transformed into delicate gongs.
- Glass lamp shades, crystal glasses, sheet glass—drilled, suspended, and gently struck.

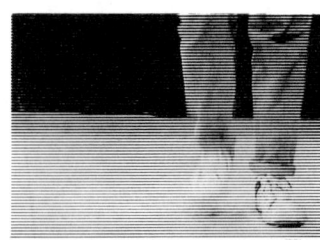

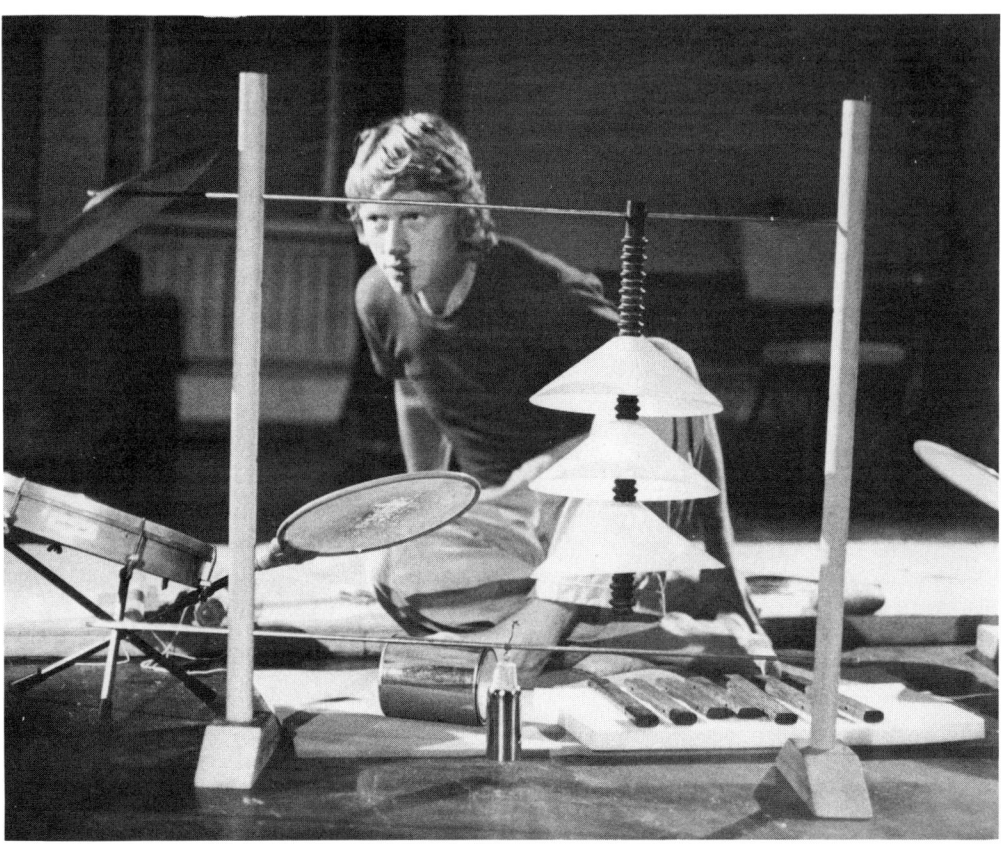

Pottery/stone

- Mixing bowls, dessert bowls, fruit bowls, flower pots, Chinese rice and soup bowls, and any other sorts of porcelain. These, like tins and bottles, can be arranged in a circle or semi-circle at floor level, on a pad of foam, with or without water. Rice bowls played with chopsticks ping well!
- Some hard varieties of stone ring, but finding a source may not be easy.
- Small hand-sized stones, paired, can be good for clicking sounds.

These materials remain lifeless until assembled with imagination and activated with the right sorts of beaters—hard, medium, or soft. Try rubber balls (Superballs are good for some materials) glued onto lengths of dowel or cane. The aim is to minimize contact sound and optimize pitch and tone quality.

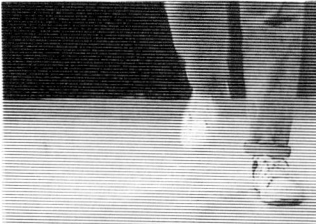

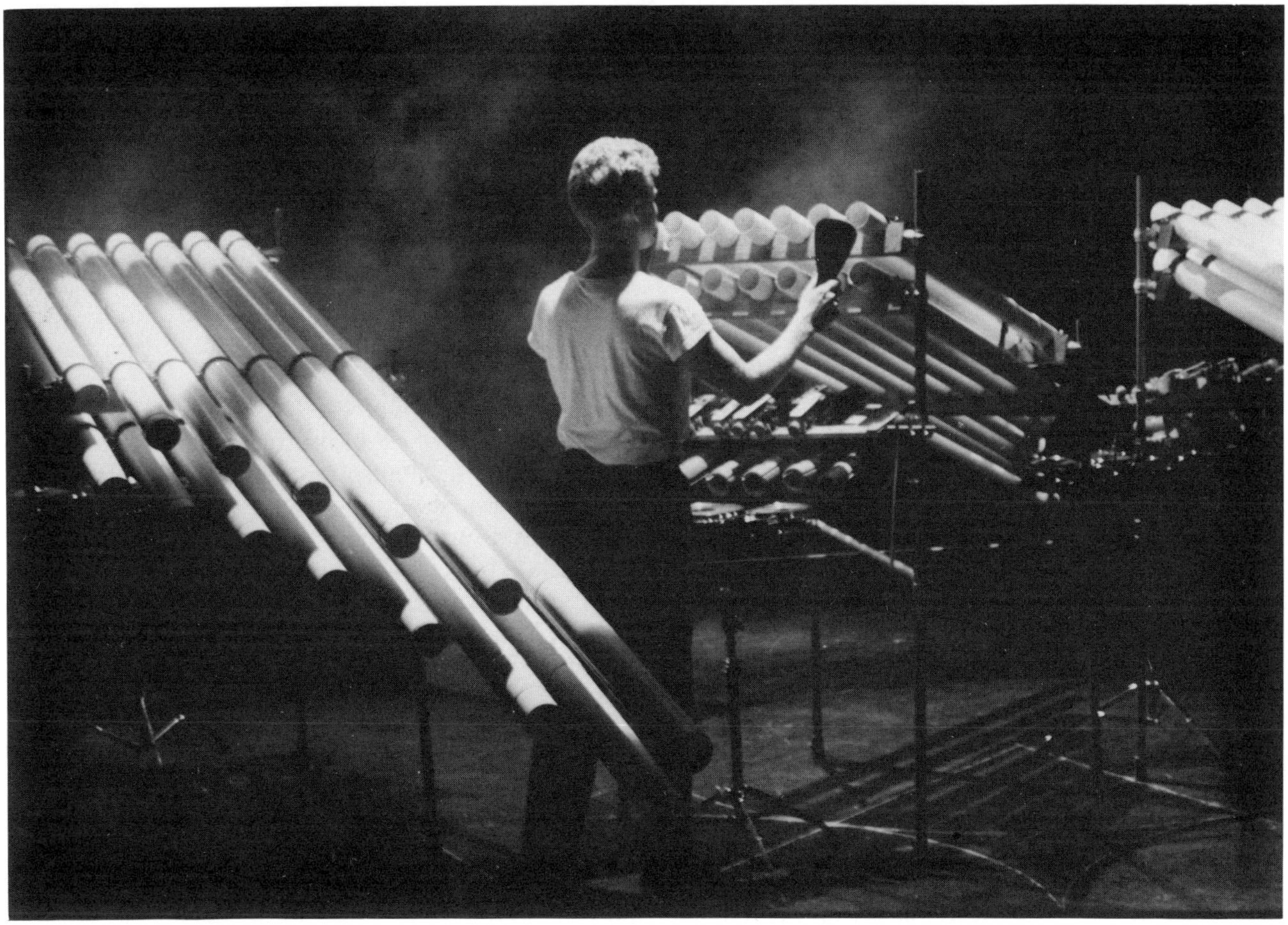

If you are interested in following up further sources for homemade instruments, there are some very good books available. Try your local library for:

Experimental Musical Instruments, an excellent quarterly magazine. Current and back issues are available by back order from EMI, P.O. Box 784, Nicasio, CA 94946, United States.

Genesis of a Music, by Harry Partch, Da Capo Press Inc,, New York. This is an absolute treasure of music history, philosophy, "just" and other tuning systems, instrument invention and anecdotes.

Vibrations, by David Sawyer, Cambridge University Press, England

Sound Designs: A Handbook of Musical Instrument Building, by Reinhold Banek and Jon Scoville, Ten Speed Press, California.

And if you want more information about any of the From Scratch instruments, write to Phil Dadson, P.O. Box 66060, Beachhaven, Auckland 1310, New Zealand.

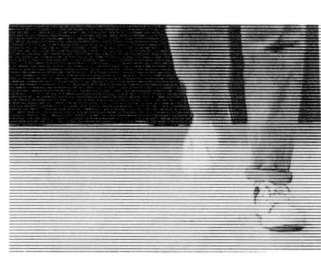

FROM SCRATCH RECORDINGS

- *From Scratch Perform Rhythm Works.* L.P. 1979
  "Out-In." Tuned PVC pipes, metal chimes, drums, voices.
  "Drumwheel," as above plus drum tubes, slit gongs, brake drums, growlers, snare drum, and bells. Performed by Geoff Chapple, Philip Dadson, Wayne Laird, Don McGlashan, Gary Wain. Devised by Philip Dadson.
- *3 Pieces from Gung Ho 1, 2, 3D.* E.P. 1982 (out of print)
- *"Gung Ho 1, 2, 3D."* L.P. (Flying Nun 085) 1987. (A remix of the complete work recorded 1981.) Tuned PVC pipes, metal chimes, drums, spun drones. Performed by Geoff Chapple, Philip Dadson, Wayne Laird, Don McGlashan. Devised by Philip Dadson.
- *From Scratch: Drum/Sing and Pacific 3, 2, 1, Zero Part 1.* L.P. (Flying Nun 0410) 1984.
  "Drum/Sing." Tuned PVC pipes, chimes, bamboos, drums, handbells, spun drones. Performed and devised by Philip Dadson, Wayne Laird, Don McGlashan.
  "Pacific 3, 2, 1, Zero Part 1." Tuned PVC pipes, chimes, drums, cymbals, voices, trom tubes, spun drones, rattle-jackets, biscuit tins. Performed and devised by Philip Dadson, Wayne Laird, and Don McGlashan, with thanks to Geoff Chapple.
- *Drum/Sing.* 16-mm film collaboration, with filmmaker Gregor Nicholas. 1st Prize, Film as Art, 28th American Film Festival, New York, 1986. Performed/devised as above. Available on VHS video, PAL, and NTSC. 20'
- *Pacific 3, 2, 1, Zero, Parts 1 and 2.* Live at Auckland Girls Grammar Gymnasium. Cassette. 1986. Part 1, as above. Part 2. Aluminum pipes tossed and struck, tuned wood and metal claves, voices, tuned-tongue PVCs, 3 trombones, 3 saxophones, and bamboo seed-poles. Philip Dadson, Ben Harrop, Alison Henry, Wayne Laird, Joshna La Trobe, Diipali Linwood, Don McGlashan, Deborah Maud, Nicola May, Aldas Palubinskas, Peter Scholes, and Kim Wesney. Devised by Philip Dadson.
- *Songs for Heros.* CD and cassette (Rattle Records, RAT D002 & RAT C002 1991). Zitherum drones, PVC pipe and drum stations, vocals, hand-clapping, tone-trees, piano-horn, soprano saxophone, and voice harmonics. Performed by Philip Dadson, Neville Hall, James McCarthy and Walter Muller. Devised by Philip Dadson.
- *Pacific 3, 2, 1, Zero.* 16-mm film collaboration with filmmaker Gregor Nicholas, 1993 (Grand Prix, Cannes/Midem, 1994). Performed by Philip Dadson, Wayne Laird, and James McCarthy. Devised as above. Available on (S)VHS video, PAL and NTSC. 23'
- *Fax-to-Paris.* Part of the Compilation CD and cassette, *"Different Tracks"* (RAT D003). 1992. Tone-trees, tuned drums, hand-clapping, and vocals. Performed by Philip Dadson, Neville Hall, James McCarthy, and Walter Muller. Devised by Philip Dadson.
- *From Scratch: Pacific 3, 2, 1, Zero: Eye-Drum,* CD and cassette. (Kiwi-Pacific International CD SLC-236) 1995. "Pacific 3,2,1, Zero"—(new digital recording) as above. "Eye-Drum"—eye drum stations, gongs, bass pipes, PVC pipes and bass drums, sliding sleeve percussion, membrane drones, sopr' sax, song-stones, gold pans, zitherum drone, tuned-tongue bells, and voices. Performed by Philip Dadson, Neville Hall, James McCarthy and Walter Muller. Devised by Philip Dadson.

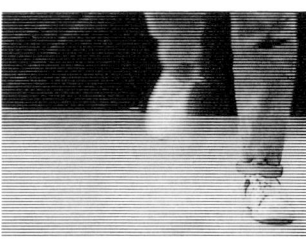